PRAISE FOR THE BOOK *THE INSIGHTFUL*

"*The Insightful Body* is much more than a book… It is a step-by-step course for therapists, offering a range of processes and insights, to facilitate communication with the wisdom of their clients' bodies."

—*Bruce Burger, MA, RPP, founder of Heartwood Institute and author of* Esoteric Anatomy: The Body as Consciousness

"This manual is a wonderful resource for practitioners seeking to develop or improve skills in bringing about healing, through the integration of the language of evocative words with the language of gentle touch. Its detailed descriptions of a wide range of techniques and of protocols with which to structure sessions makes it immediately relevant. Julie's appreciation of the difficulty one can feel venturing into this domain for the first time is especially helpful."

—*Mike Brenner, integrative practitioner*

"Each day as a practitioner I am faced with the challenge of trying to understand, communicate, and make a difference with each of my clients… Julie has given me the tools to better understand myself, know which type of communicator I am and help me correspond with my clients. Her advice is well-written, comprehensive and easy to implement… After reading her book, I feel that I have the necessary tools to get beyond the communication barriers and treat the patient much more effectively."

—*Dr. Kerry D'Ambrogio DOM, AP, DO-MTP, PT, Doctor of Oriental Medicine, osteopath, physical therapist, and founder of Therapeutic Systems Incorporated*

"As human consciousness evolves, we continue to develop greater and greater awareness of the mind/body connection, and the many ways in which our bodies mirror our emotions and thought patterns. In *The Insightful Body*, Julie McKay has given us a clear, insightful, ground-breaking roadmap for learning the language of the body, and listening to all it has to teach us about ourselves, and about those we seek to help. It is an invaluable contribution to the literature on physical and expressive therapies."

—*John E. Welshons, author of* One Soul, One Love, One Heart *and* Awakening from Grief

"This book takes you beyond communicating with your client to true interaction with body, mind and spirit. I learned from this book, and because of it will continue to learn more with each interaction with my clients. Improved communication, improved outcomes, continued learning and growth for both the client and the bodyworker… Fabulous! This is what the therapeutic relationship is all about!"

—*Jean Wible, RN, BSN, NCTMB, LMT, HTCP, author of* Pharmacology for Massage Therapy *and* Drug Handbook for Massage Therapists

"A great gift to the therapeutic community. Julie has created a Rosetta Stone for healers to translate the wisdom which is inherent yet unique in every person's body. This wonderful resource has something for every therapist of varying disciplines and skill levels. It is full of well-described techniques to start using right away."

—Maria C.S. Gabelberger, Psy.D, licensed clinical psychologist
and Ericksonian hypnotherapist in private practice

"Julie McKay's *The Insightful Body* is an essential guide that proves that through communication and understanding we can all be the beneficiaries of powerful and healthy human connections. A must read for any therapist who aspires to unconditionally and effectively support their client's journey towards self discovery."

—Jean E. Thompson, chiropractor

"This book is a must have for any therapist who wants to facilitate the awakening of the perfect healer in each of their patients/clients."

—Perci Kotter, LMT, certified Zero Balancing practitioner

PRAISE FOR SOMACENTRIC DIALOGUING WORKSHOPS

"A great resource to develop new skills to help clients get in touch with and move through resistant difficulties."

—Denise Supik, psychologist

"This is a wonderful opportunity to gain very down-to-earth-type questions that encourage clients to engage their own healing. Takes the 'mystery' out of how to ask questions."

—Kathleen Abrams, speech-language pathologist

"Adds another meaty piece to my repertoire of methods to enhance the work I do. This enriches the experience and provides more concrete ways for clients to be with their bodies more easily. Thank you!"

—Betsy Granek, RN, massage therapist

"This is a practical, nuts-and-bolts workshop that has broadened my understanding and knowledge of how to get beyond the head and into the body. I am going back to work with a truly different outlook in how to engage!"

—Dolores Arroyo, occupational therapist

THE INSIGHTFUL BODY

of related interest

Relating to Clients
The Therapeutic Relationship for Complementary Therapists
Su Fox
ISBN 978 1 84310 615 9

Meet Your Body
CORE Bodywork and Rolfing Tools to Release Bodymindcore Trauma
Noah Karrasch
Illustrated by Lovella Lindsey
ISBN 978 1 84819 016 0

You Are How You Move
Experiential Chi Kung
Ged Sumner
ISBN 978 1 84819 014 6

Body Intelligence
Creating a New Environment
Second Edition
Ged Sumner
ISBN 978 1 84819 026 9

Curves, Twists and Bends
A Practical Guide to Pilates for Scoliosis
Annette Wellings and Alan Herdman
ISBN 978 1 84819 025 2

The
Insightful
Body

HEALING

WITH SOMACENTRIC

DIALOGUING

JULIE MCKAY

SINGING DRAGON
LONDON AND PHILADELPHIA

Author photo by Giovanni Pescetto © Julie McKay 2010
protection illustrations © Thomas B. Crossan, IV 2010
Llama, security guard, bodyguard, owl, balloons, resistance, and.
Julie, double arrows, compass, plane ticket, and calendar illustrations © Julie McKay. 2010

First published in 2010
by Singing Dragon
an imprint of Jessica Kingsley Publishers
116 Pentonville Road
London N1 9JB, UK
and
400 Market Street, Suite 400
Philadelphia, PA 19106, USA

www.singing-dragon.com

Copyright © Julie McKay 2010

Library of Congress Cataloging in Publication Data
A CIP catalog record for this book is available from the Library of Congress

British Library Cataloguing in Publication Data
A CIP catalogue record for this book is available from the British Library

ISBN 978 1 84819 030 6

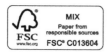

"There is more wisdom in your body
than in your deepest philosophy."

—Friedrich Nietzsche

"It's not so much that there are mysteries in the body,
it's just you can't hear what the body is saying."

—Kelly Russell

Contents

Acknowledgments

Teachers come in many forms and at various times.

I want to thank my clients who have taught me many things through their sessions. During sessions, I have the honor of watching incredible transformations happen. Afterward, clients often thank me with tears in their eyes. They tell me how profound their realizations are. I thank them for coming and tell them that I am glad to be of service. After they leave, I close the door and wonder for a few minutes, "How did that happen?" Sometimes I am just as amazed as my clients are, and I learn from their sessions.

Particularly influential teachers I would like to thank for their inspiration are Bruce Burger, Rhonda Hilyer, Tim Hutton, Howard Loomis Jr., Elizabeth Wiley, and Patrick Woods.

Thank you to my colleagues who inspired me to create workshops about SomaCentric Dialoguing so they could learn it. And to Kelly and my friends for believing in me and continually encouraging me as I diligently put all this down on paper. Thank you to Barbara, Carrie, Dave, Mike, and Perci for your editing and feedback. And to all at Jessica Kingsley Publishers for valuing my work and helping this to be a delightful experience.

And most of all I want to acknowledge what I learned from my mother. Two years before she passed away, we were talking about the work that I do. She wanted to know more and understand better how I help people. I recounted to her the following story.

At six years old, I got a new, shiny, green bike for Christmas. It had a banana seat and streamers on the wide handle bars and no training wheels. It was a previously owned and well-loved bike, but new to me, and that was all that mattered. The following spring I rode it on the sidewalk in front of our house. I was still a little wobbly, with no training wheels to steady me, and I happened to fall off. My mother's sharp ears recognized that something was amiss, and she came to brush me off.

She sat on the sidewalk with me and asked me where I hurt. I pointed to the large red scrape and told her my knee hurt. She gave it special medicine, a mother's kiss. Next, Mom told me something that would have a profound effect upon my life, although I would not realize it until decades later. She told me to tell my knee that it was okay. She helped me tell my knee that I had not broken anything. I told my knee it was only scraped, and we would take care of it. Mom told me that the pain was my knee trying to get my brain's attention so I would take care of it. Mom suggested that I also make my knee feel nice and soft like a marshmallow, thus, as I have realized years later, helping it to relax.

We sat there a few more minutes. I told my knee that it could be soft like a marshmallow and stop hurting. I had gotten the message and thanked it for getting my attention to let me know that there was a problem. After Mom brushed off the dirt and hugged me, I got back on my bike with a smile and no pain.

Thanks, Mom, for teaching me how to pay attention to and talk with my body.

Introduction

For ten years, I had been a professional bodyworker when bodywork came to my rescue. One morning I started to experience unusual sensations. It started as an itching, then a burning, then an unusual pain. I thought I had slipped a disc in my back, or perhaps it was a major yeast infection. I did not want to subject myself to the allopathic medical community, especially since I did not have health insurance and it would create a financial nightmare to diagnose my problem.

I turned to my extensive community of fellow therapists for help. I agreed with my chiropractor that I would get an MRI if I experienced certain neurological problems. Although my care was provided by some of the top therapists in the area, none of them knew the exact source of my problems. I experienced pain 24 hours a day, seven days a week.

It took 18 months of consistent, chiropractic care, massage therapy, acupuncture, and other forms of bodywork to start to get some relief. I tried deep-tissue massage, neuromuscular therapy, myofascial, Rolfing, Zero Balancing, Network Spinal Analysis, BioValent Systems, acupuncture, nutrition, and, of course, CranioSacral Therapy and SomatoEmotional Release.

I examined my life to see if there was a lesson that I needed to learn. I sat with my unremitting pain to try to find the lesson behind it. Surely I was supposed to learn something from this ordeal. An ordeal it was—some days the moment I became conscious, emerging from sleep, I would wake up in pain. I went to work regardless of the excruciating pain. Some days it was a little better, not as intense. Other days I would come home thoroughly exhausted, even if it had not been a long work day.

The pain exhausted me. Not knowing what was going on exhausted me. Not knowing how to take care of the pain exhausted me. Not knowing when it would get better became depressing.

Therapists and friends would ask me what my pain felt like or how my pain was. I had a difficult time answering. I could tell them at any given time when and where I felt it. The difficulty lay in how to describe what the pain, what the "It," felt like. Over time I realized there was more to "It" than pain.

I finally realized the lesson of my pain when I reflected about what to write for this introduction. The lesson was to learn fully that pain means many things to many people and to teach others how to help determine how their clients can clearly articulate what they feel. Pain may be described as an ache by one person or a stiff sensation by another. Pain has many descriptions: sharp, dull, sore, tiring, stabbing, big, pointed, nagging, excruciating, heavy, etc.

Let me describe my pain to you, so you can decide how to best label "It." First, It started in my groin with a tingly sensation. Initially, I thought I might have a yeast infection; but over the next couple of days and being unresponsive to high-powered yeast-infection medication, It went down the inside of my thighs and the backs of my calves to the soles of my feet. Over the first weeks, It continued to move throughout my legs and travel up to my back. As time progressed, the tingly sensation got stronger and more uncomfortable, starting to feel like prickly heat. After a few months, wearing jeans was uncomfortable because the fabric was too rough and scratchy. I could only tolerate It with the softest and loosest clothes. It caused the sensation of a "belt" that went around the lower part of my rib cage, all the way around my torso with this "pain." My stomach started to react with heartburn-type symptoms. It continued to expand to my hands and my arms. It did not follow any particular region or area of my body; It did not stick to any dermatomes.

To work hurt. My legs bothered me particularly when I sat. My hands bothered me when I stayed in one position for a long time. As a CranioSacral Therapist, I generally have to sit still for minutes on end. This posture exacerbated my It, my pain. I realized as the months wore on that movement was my ally.

Over time, I realized that It felt kind of familiar. It reminded me of something I had previously experienced. Finally, I had some words to describe It more accurately. Rather than describe the sensation as pain, It felt like this: picture yourself going outside, in the late fall, without gloves on, walking to the corner store or taking out the garbage. You come back inside and rub your hands together because they are cold and hurt. This feeling is not quite a pain, not in the truest sense. Your hands have a hot, irritated, pin-prickly sensation, maybe with a swelling feeling. They hurt; there is a sort of pain but not excruciating. That is what my It feels like. That is what my "pain" felt like.

If I had told you I had pain in my legs, would you have thought of that description? Probably not. All the therapists I have worked with did not have that image when I told them I had pain or discomfort.

I have lived with It and have been healing It over two years. I have realized that when asked "Are you in pain?" I have to answer the question honestly, "No, I am not in pain." If asked if I am uncomfortable, I answer, "Yes, I am in a lot of discomfort." Thus, when asked to describe my pain, I have a difficult time because It truly is not pain but is uncomfortable.

I previously said "My back is bothering me" to identify that I was uncomfortable and did not feel physically well. I used this phrase because I thought that my It, my pain, was from a slipped disc. Months of chiropractic care were helpful, but my not healing proved to my chiropractors and me that a slipped or bulging disc was not the cause of my problem.

Once I realized that the problem was not my back, I had a difficult time articulating how I felt. I once said to a concerned friend, "Well, my hot, prickly, tingly, weird, strange as-yet-unidentified nerve-like but not neuralgic pain is bothering me again." Because I wanted to communicate that I was in discomfort but knew full well the source was not my back and also did not want to mislead my therapists, I could not say, "My back is bothering me." The best I came up to describe It was "I'm having a flare-up."

My struggle made me think about those who suffer from chronic, sometimes vague, or difficult-to-identify pain conditions such as fibromyalgia, chronic fatigue, Epstein-Barr syndrome, and Lyme disease. Those who suffer from these and other conditions find it difficult to describe how and what they experience to their family, friends, and most importantly to their health-care providers. The situation is exacerbated with conditions like rheumatoid arthritis or multiple sclerosis, where the symptomology is broad and varied. Each person has her own list, similar to but not exactly like the list of the next person with the same diagnosis.

It takes a very skilled practitioner to be able to ask simple questions to help a person specifically articulate what is being experienced. I got lucky, lucky that I knew what to ask of myself. I knew how to describe the patterns and what It felt like to me. My experience as a practitioner helped me tell my therapists what I experienced. My articulate words and the therapists' hands allowed them to tell me, "It's not your back that is your problem." It took 18 months finally to realize that abdominal fascial restrictions, from a thrown phone book hitting me in the stomach, caused It, my pain.

My lesson, taught by It, was to realize that sometimes even highly skilled therapists do not know how or what to ask their client, in order for their client to articulate what he is experiencing. The words a client uses are often broad and vague because of the uncertainty and muddle of emotions he is experiencing. The words that therapists use are often vague, general, and generic. Often the therapist repeats back what the client has said with a tone of assumed understanding and knowing.

Do you understand what you really say to your client?

Do you easily understand what your client communicates to you?

Do you understand what your client tells you when she wants to know about how you are, before she tells you about how she is?

Do you understand what happens when you ask "How does your leg feel?" but your client is not able to articulate anything?

Would you like to have clear communication with your client? Your job would be easier if you were able to distinguish between an ache and a stabbing pain. These different words have different connotations and mean different things from a physiological standpoint.

In this book, you will learn about how to answer these questions with the SomaCentric Dialoguing System.[1] I always paid attention to the importance of communication when I was in various leadership, sales, and management positions during the last 20 years. As a therapist, I have spent over ten years refining the techniques that I use with clients. From a variety of therapies and personal insights, I have learned how to identify what language my client speaks, so that I can more effectively communicate with her. I help clients learn how to become more aware of the messages their bodies try to communicate to them, which creates a deeper level of healing.

I quickly realized, after providing some tutoring and being asked to teach workshops about dialoguing and helping clients improve their body-centered awareness, that nowhere are these concepts collected together in one place. I realized that I have used concepts that I had learned from over ten different therapies or communication styles. Over time, I changed and improved upon what I originally learned by blending certain aspects of these concepts. Doing so has allowed me to help my clients more thoroughly.

For example, the "Just Because" and "Surgery Prep" techniques presented in this book are my original creations. Other techniques are modifications of widely used fundamentals in the realm of working with body consciousness, although as I have presented them, they have my own fingerprints on them, based on what has worked for me in my treatment room.

I present to you SomaCentric Dialoguing, a system to help you, the therapist, determine what your client is trying to say and how to help her get in touch with her body. With SomaCentric Dialoguing, your sessions will go beyond your client's expectations to become life transformations. SomaCentric Dialoguing[1] will allow you to help your client articulate what her "It" is and the message that her body and her "It" have for her.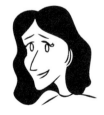

---

1   The terms SomaCentric Dialoguing and SomaCentric Dialoguing System are trademarked by Julie McKay. Therapists may use these terms only upon successful completion of prescribed instruction on SomaCentric Dialoguing as presented by Julie McKay or The CLEAR Institute™.

1 *What It Is All About*

Over the last 18 years, ten years as a manual therapist and the previous eight years doing other health-related work, I have paid close attention to what my clients really say. I first learned about dialoguing through my training as a certified Bach practitioner and as a polarity therapist. After I took SomatoEmotional Release® (SER) classes, I realized that a lot could be added to the classes or explored but was not taught (for various reasons). Over the years, I have incorporated into my SER sessions these other concepts and tools that are extremely helpful.

My work in communication with clients has been strongly influenced by the work of Rhonda Hilyer, author of *Success Signals*; Dawna Markova, PhD, author of *The Open Mind: Exploring the 6 Patterns of Natural Intelligence*; and Rick Carson, author of *Taming Your Gremlin*.

During the last year, many therapists who have attended my CranioSacral Therapy study groups asked me to develop a specific class about how SER therapists can dialogue more effectively with their clients. While creating this class, I quickly realized that much of this material was also pertinent for therapists who have not learned CranioSacral Therapy and SomatoEmotional Release. I want to be very clear that I am not teaching CranioSacral Therapy, SomatoEmotional Release, or any form of psychotherapy. You must determine what material is appropriate to use in your practice and with your clients according to your license and scope of practice.[1]

---

1   Any tools or techniques presented in this book are intended for your informational benefit only and are not a substitute for professional medical treatment or training. You must practice in accordance with your professional certification or license and not employ techniques that are outside your professional scope of practice.

SomaCentric Dialoguing is a multifaceted, body-centered (or somacentric) system. It teaches you how to go beyond conversing with your client to facilitate her own healing process. You will help her do this by bringing her own awarenesses to consciousness, rather than just by removing physical symptoms and "fixing" her problem. SomaCentric Dialoguing is about many things. The unifying aspect of this system, book, and the SomaCentric Dialoguing workshops is how to learn the language that your client speaks, so you can optimally communicate with her, enhance her body-centered awareness and integration, and help her in her healing journey.

SomaCentric Dialoguing is an adjunctive therapy. It is not psychotherapy, nor is it a primary therapy. Rather, it is designed to be used *in conjunction* with other therapies, such as bodywork, acupuncture, or "talk therapies." SomaCentric Dialoguing is designed to help other therapies be more effective and more thorough than they might be on their own.

Throughout this book, you will come across some simple—but not simplistic—concepts. When they are put together, they have profound results. The SomaCentric Dialoguing system teaches you how to get your clients to say, "My therapist really understands me!"

You will become aware from start to finish how to:

- identify what communication style and processing language your client speaks

- refine your dialoguing vocabulary

- ask more effective questions

- create a thorough session

- help your client become more aware of what occurs in her body and be an active participant in her healing

I call all this SomaCentric Dialoguing because the focus is to help the client center (centric) her awareness on her body (soma) and dialogue with her body. Therapists speak or dialogue with their client's body, not only her mind. This system is designed for any person, health-care practitioner, acupuncturist, bodyworker, physical therapist, occupational therapist, social worker, psychologist, movement therapist, and medical doctor who cares about what happens with her client/patient. When you are able to identify what language your client speaks and ask broad, open-ended questions, you will quickly get more information than you have before.

You will read about

- how to ask more effective questions

- what words to use and what words to avoid for optimal results

- how to go beyond just talking or conversing with your client and really carry on a dialogue with your client

- how to empower your client with Wiggle Words

- how to focus your client's body-awareness

- what techniques will start a session and end a session and what to do if you get stuck

- what techniques explore specific problems

- what techniques to teach clients for self-care

With a more refined vocabulary and easy-to-use techniques, you can help your client effectively let go of holding patterns and pain in his body. These effective techniques result in core physical, mental, and emotional healing. When you help your client dialogue with his body, he can heal more completely and deeply.[2]

This book and the SomaCentric Dialoguing workshops are designed to take you, the therapist, regardless of dialoguing experience, to a higher and more refined level of dialoguing with your clients. They are designed to take you beyond conversing with your client, to be able to engage your client with the language that she speaks. Throughout this book, I will present ideas and concepts. Some of them you may already use, while some may be new or unfamiliar. Some items may not work with your style of therapy. I invite you to take what you like and incorporate them into your session; leave the other material on the page for another time.

You will get the most from this book if you read it from start to finish. That said, feel free to jump from chapter to chapter, depending upon what catches your interest. Individual chapters can be read independently of the previous chapter(s). If you do this and find a concept or technique referred to with which you are unfamiliar, just go back and read the appropriate chapter.

Real-life examples of client sessions are used throughout the book. They are taken straight out of my treatment room. I use them to help you better understand the techniques and to help you get a clearer idea of what SomaCentric Dialoguing is about. The names of clients have been changed to protect the identity of the person. I encourage you to think about your clients and their struggles as you read these client sessions and learn about the communication and processing languages. It is my hope that you will find a technique or combination of techniques to help your client. Get creative with how these can be used.

Collected together in one of the last chapters, "Techniques Review," are all the session information and techniques in an easy-to-use reference format:

---

2   Throughout the text, you will notice that I alternate the use of masculine and feminine pronouns to refer to a client. The use of "he" or "she" in any given concept or section does not imply any gender bias or that I have seen more clients of one sex or another with any particular problem. Of course, anywhere a client is "named," the name has been changed to protect the identity of the individual.

- structure for a typical SomaCentric Dialoguing session

- how to frame the session, at the start and at the finish

- session opening and closing recitation

- how to get started

- how to resolve resistance

- session techniques

- self-care/homework techniques for clients

- a synopsis of communication styles and processing languages

You will find a brief synopsis of the main intent of each technique along with the basic instructions. I have done this so you can easily refer to it by simply propping open the book and have it close at hand during your sessions. And four of these techniques are appropriate for your clients to use as self-care or homework.

Some chapters have accompanying exercises designed to help expand your thinking and awareness of presented concepts. I highly encourage you to use the space provided to pencil in your own responses. There are no "right" or "wrong" answers, but some will be more true and accurate to the concept discussed. In chapter 16, "Exercise Review," you will find the exercises collected together with responses from SomaCentric Dialoguing workshop participants. I encourage you to use these to expand your dialoguing vocabulary.

The discussions throughout mention manual therapy and physical contact with clients. However, the material can and often does apply even if you are a nontouch therapist. If you are not a manual therapist and you read something like "take your hands off your client and take a deep breath," just disregard the part about taking your hands off. Simply "take a deep breath." It is the concept of what is being presented that I want you to understand and perhaps incorporate into your sessions, if appropriate.

You will discover very effective dialoguing techniques to help your client resolve problems. These effective techniques result in core physical, mental, and emotional healing. When you are able to speak the same language as your client, you can improve general rapport and interactions. This will help you improve your client-history intake and gather more information. Use your client's language to help her become more aware of what is going on in her body. This helps her more effectively let go of holding patterns, stored emotions, and pain in her body, which make sessions more effective. When you learn to speak your client's language, you will understand her better.

2 Creating and Holding a Safe Space

Be Here Now

Be Here Now is the title of one of Ram Dass's books. It is quoted often for a variety of reasons. I use it here to help illustrate how to create and hold a safe space for clients.

It is of primary importance that your client feels safe. When you, the therapist, hold a space in safety, your client can feel safe more easily, and this feeling enhances his awareness of what is happening inside of him. These concepts are ones we have heard repeatedly. I present them because it is always helpful to be reminded of them. I invite you to find how you can more fully embody these concepts.

As a therapist, to hold a safe space a few fundamentals need to happen.

YOU NEED TO BE

1. Yourself

Be fully yourself. You can only be one person, and that is your incredible you. Yes, you are incredible. There is something about you that allows your client to place her vulnerable self in your hands. The only way you can do her justice is to be fully yourself, not someone else, nor the person you think she wants you to be.

If you try to be someone or something other than who you are, the client's subconscious will know that something is not genuine or authentic. It may go unmentioned, but her own inner knowing or intuition will send off warning signals that she may not be safe. It is best for all if you simply be yourself.

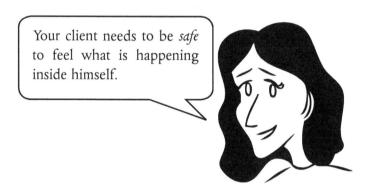

Your client needs to be *safe* to feel what is happening inside himself.

2. Focused

Pay full attention to your client. Do not daydream or think about your shopping list. It is okay to admit to yourself that you have done that. I know I have. When my focus drifts, I catch myself and bring my focus back to my client and the session. The quicker you can identify when your focus has drifted and bring yourself back to the client, the better the session will be.

3. Grounded

Keep both feet on the floor. Bring energy into your body through your feet and your crown. This helps to balance the energy coming from above and from below you. When you stay grounded, you can pay better attention to your body mechanics. You can stay more relaxed. You can be more emotionally neutral. There are many wonderful books and audio CDs about grounding, so I will not go into detail. If you need a good resource, I suggest Suzanne Scurlock-Durana's "Healing from the Core" books, audio CDs, and classes.

YOU NEED TO BE HERE

Present

Be present in each moment. To be present fully for your client, you also need to be present fully in your own body. Be in the session room with your attention on your client. If you have to step out of the room for any reason—while she undresses, while you wash your hands, etc.—make sure you keep your mental attention on your client. Otherwise, it is easy to get distracted, such as by a comment from someone passing you in the hall. Or you might be reminded of something you need to do after work. When you then go back into your treatment room, your attention may still linger on the distraction rather than being fully focused on your client. When you stay focused, it is easier to remain present with your client.

YOU NEED TO BE HERE NOW
In the moment

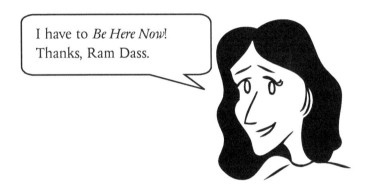

I have to *Be Here Now*! Thanks, Ram Dass.

Be in the current moment, current time. Avoid the mental shopping lists, daydreaming, or mental arguments with the landlord or person who cut you off while you were driving to work. Check in with yourself if you catch your mind wandering off. If necessary, take your hands off your client, and take a deep breath to bring yourself back to what is happening in front of you.

Why is all this important?

It can be intimidating for your client to consider getting in touch with what is going on inside him. The world outside is already scary for many. Your client's inner world might be an even more terrifying place. If you are unsettled or not present, your client will pick up on it, and he may not feel safe. He may not feel that you can be present with him when he experiences his worst. If the environment of the treatment room is perceived as uncomfortable, threatening, or unsafe, then the amount of energy needed to cope with what is stored inside can be overwhelming. The energy necessary to work with what is inside may not be available to your client. Because he does not feel safe, he may not then be willing to "go there." It is your job as a therapist to create a safe place where your client can easily use whatever resources he has to access in his own body to help facilitate his own healing process.

TO CREATE A SAFE SPACE

To create a safe space I have to show up fully. To do this I have to:

- be within myself

- be fully present

- be in the moment, current time (not elsewhere—a mental shopping list or argument or daydream)

This safe space must be maintained throughout the session. As you will learn, sometimes it will be necessary for the client to create a safe space for herself. Later in chapter 10, "Getting Started," I explain how to have your client use the Safe Space Conversation to help her resolve issues that come up or that are hindering her therapy.

3 *Key Concepts*

Before I go any further, I want to discuss some important concepts that you need to heed and incorporate. These key concepts can be crucial to help hold a safe space and to keep the session focused on the client's intentions. Topics covered include your role as facilitator, the difference between understanding and knowledge, the cause of problems, the importance of recognizing indicators, and the problems of a client's saying "you" versus "I" and of "then" versus "now." These will be briefly discussed to help set the framework for a SomaCentric Dialoguing session. There are two very good books that I highly encourage you to read, both of which go into more detail about these and other similar topics. They are *Lessons from the Sessions* by Don Ash, PT, CST-D, and *The Educated Heart* by Nina McIntosh.

FACILITATOR

Your role as a therapist doing SomaCentric Dialoguing is that of the facilitator. A facilitator is defined by *The American Heritage® Dictionary of the English Language* as one whose role it is to make something easier. When you apply that definition to SomaCentric Dialoguing, your role is to make it easier for your client to become aware of what her body wants her to know. Your job is to help your client gain a better awareness of what is going on in a given situation and what message(s) her body has for her; you assist or make it easier for her to be in an emotional place that may be scary or difficult for her and help your client get in tune with what is going on in her body.

Because SomaCentric Dialoguing is not psychotherapy, it is important to avoid analyzing or determining the meaning of a client's situation or problem. It is not your job to interpret what or why something is or is not happening. *You are solely a facilitator.* It is not part of your role in SomaCentric Dialoguing to draw any conclusions from the session. SomaCentric Dialoguing is about having the client be in touch with what is happening with her body so that *she* can interpret what something means. Your client, through SomaCentric Dialoguing, figures out the "whys" of her situation and how it applies to her life.

One of my favorite analogies about the role of the therapist and how a SomaCentric Dialoguing session unfolds is that a session is like a painting. Your client holds the brush, and you are holding the palette of paints for her to use. Your client first puts a few brush strokes of a few colors on the canvas, then, a few more. You continue to assist by holding the paint. The image that emerges may be abstract and disjointed, similar to artwork by Picasso. The more that dialogue occurs the more that details are revealed. The abstract painting starts taking on a more impressionistic feel. Perhaps it becomes a Monet or a Seurat. More color and detail are created by the increased depth of the session. As your client becomes more aware and better understands the message(s) her body has, the painting now transforms into one of greater clarity, a painting from the Renaissance period, perhaps a Botticelli. By now, the finer details have all been filled in, and a complete scene has unfolded before you and your client. While you hold the paints, your client has revealed what her body wanted her to realize.

A couple of other analogies that are fun to think of are the following:

> You and your client drive in a car. Your client is behind the wheel, while you hold the map. You can only give help when your client asks for guidance.

> You are listening to a book being read aloud, a mystery novel. The author and reader of the book is your client. You patiently wait to find out what happens as your client tells you the tale.

And sometimes your role of therapist as facilitator is one who is there to "sit in the mud" with your client. The situation may feel bleak and grim, with your client stuck in the mud. The only thing to do is just to be there with her, sitting in the mud. Your presence there with her in the mud is just to assure her that she is not alone. Your role as facilitator is to witness her process nonverbally and just be with her.

Your job is to help your client get a better awareness of:
- what is going on
- what messages her body has for her
- what the scary places in her life are

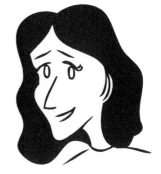

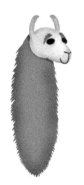

It is your job to have your client:
- determine meanings
- interpret connections
- draw conclusions

CAUSES OF PROBLEMS

Problems, like people, come in many different shapes and sizes. The causes of problems come from four fundamental stresses: physical, emotional/mental, nutritional, and spiritual. SomaCentric Dialoguing focuses on the physical and emotional stresses, even though there may be components involved that are nutritionally or spiritually based. It is not always necessary to know the cause of the stress immediately.

Sometimes the cause of the problem or stress is not revealed until the very end of a session. Sometimes you, as the therapist, may think you know the obvious problem and want to shout out, "Look there! There's the problem!" What you know, through your own (mis)perceptions and filters, may not be the root of the problem; it may be part of or similar to the problem. As the therapist, you facilitate the session and need to let your client be in the driver's seat.

While it is not necessary to know from the start the reason for the problem to do an effective SomaCentric Dialoguing session, it is helpful information for you, as the therapist, to have filled in the background with what might be a possible cause of the problem.

Reasons for problems include physical or emotional neglect, inducement by an external source, overuse or misuse of a body part, learned behavior, unacknowledged messages from the body, and resonance, all of which can come from or can create physical or emotional stresses. For example, neglect is simply not taking proper care of something. If you neglect to change the oil in your car, eventually the warning light will come on to indicate that the engine has a problem and needs to be checked.

Examples include the following:

- Wearing improper running shoes while training for a marathon (physical neglect) can cause emotional stress by knowing one is not taking care of oneself. It can also cause a physical problem by prematurely wearing down the menisci of the knees and causing pain.

- Lack of being nurtured as a child (emotional neglect) can cause emotional stress by not being able to feel connected with one's partner. It can also result in a physical problem of massive weight gain.

Induced problems often result from surgery or accidental injury. These are situations that have been placed upon or created by an external influence.

Overuse or misuse comes from use too often and too much. Repetitive motion will often cause problems of a physical nature such as carpal tunnel syndrome, temporal mandibular joint dysfunction, or a rotator cuff tear.

Learned behavior and patterns can also cause problems. Those primarily of a physical nature are related to one's posture and walk. People also will imitate facial expressions or gestures, such as shrugging a shoulder. Learned behavior can include developing a naïve mistrust or prejudice.

When the body has a message to communicate and it is not being heard, the body manifests that message as a problem. The client's body tried to get his attention quietly, but after a certain point of lack of awareness from the client, the body will start to shout a little louder, "Hey buddy! Pay attention to me! We need some help!" Sometimes, it can be as simple as a scraped knee's triggering nerve impulses up to the brain to say, "Julie just fell off her bicycle. We need some help." Sometimes, it is more dramatic with "You haven't been paying attention to your intuition telling you to eat a better balanced diet, so we're going to give you a gall bladder attack to get you to pay attention."

> ### *Causes of Problems*
>
> physical stress
>
> emotional stress
>
> nutritional neglect
>
> spiritual neglect
>
> inducement by accident or problem
>
> overuse or misuse of body part
>
> learned behavior
>
> message from the body
>
> resonance

Resonance is the last cause of problems to be mentioned. Alaya Chikly, developer of Heart Centered Therapy, gave a presentation at the International Alliance of Healthcare Practitioners' *Beyond the Dura* conference in May 2008. Alaya spoke about resonance as a possible cause of problems. I realized that I had observed a number of clients who had problems created by resonance. The term *resonance* in music means to produce a sympathetic vibration. People resonate in synchrony or harmony with each other. When two people have a shared experience, such as when a woman is pregnant, she and her husband energetically vibrate at similar frequencies. This sympathetic resonance often causes what has become known as "sympathy pains," such as when the baby kicks and Dad feels it in his own body. It is a way people stay connected with a loved one.

To stay connected with a loved one can sometimes come in a bit more dangerous package. How often have you heard a client say, "My dad had high blood pressure, and now so do I." Or "It must be in my genes because I now have breast cancer just as my mom did." Is it truly genetic? Or is it a way that part of her body wanted to maintain a connection to Mom or Dad? You may truly never know. You can certainly help your client explore why her body has chosen to manifest the cancer or high-blood pressure. It very well may be a way to stay and feel connected to a loved one.

As the cause of the problem starts to reveal itself in the session, fully allow the client to make any connections to what else is happening in her body and her life. Allow her to make the interpretations.

UNDERSTANDING AND KNOWLEDGE

> Understanding is acquired…from the totality of information intentionally learned and from personal experiencings; whereas knowledge is only the automatic remembrance of words in a certain sequence.
>
> Not only is it impossible, even with all one's desire, to give to another one's own inner understanding, formed in the course of life from the said factors, but also…there exists a law that the quality of what is perceived by anyone when another person tells him something, either for his knowledge or his understanding, depends on the quality of the data formed in the person speaking.
>
> —G. I. Gurdjieff, *Meetings with Remarkable Men*, 241

This quote from Gurdjieff is from a story he tells about some monks with whom he had an opportunity to study. The difference that Gurdjieff talks about between understanding and knowledge is an important concept in SomaCentric Dialoguing. Your clients can get more effective results when they understand the information they have gathered from a session, rather than have the knowledge of something that happened in a session. Knowledge is often repeated as a phrase or words that have some meaning, but little personal transformation comes from the reiteration of the words.

When you are able to assist your client to be aware of what is happening in his body and what his body wants him to know, then he can comprehend deeper or understand better what is important. Understanding in a session comes from somatic awareness and body perceptions. It comes when your client is able to see, hear, touch, and feel what an emotion or message is. Knowledge from a session is on a more superficial level. When a client says, "My shoulder is sore because I am too stressed," this come from a place of knowledge and very little gets resolved. He comes from a place of understanding when he tells you about how his shoulder's soreness went away once he became aware of how he is working too much—and he realized inflammation caused the soreness and his body tried to get his attention.

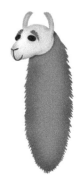

> *Understanding* is acquired—body perception, somatic awareness.

> *Knowledge* is remembrance of words in sequence—self-talk, talk therapy, redundant mental conversations.

Sometimes in a session you work at three levels—the brain, the body, and your client as a whole. Knowledge comes from and is stored in the brain. Understanding comes from and is stored by your client in her body. A phrase I sometimes hear from clients is "My doctor/psychotherapist says my problem is _____." This is knowledge. Yes, the cause and the result of the problem may be accurate, but healing is slower to occur with only knowledge. Knowledge is in the brain or head. Understanding is in the "gut" or body. Understanding comes from a gut level. Your job is to help your client get to a place of healing by helping her understand what is happening.

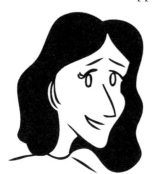

> Understanding is the "Aha!" moment.

Many times I have observed that, immediately at the end of the session, the problem, the cause, and the result were all clearly understood and able to be articulated by the client. Healing occurred of a physical, mental, and/or emotional nature. However, a week or a month later, the client would find it difficult to explain what had happened in the session. He had lost the words, even though the change in his body, the healing, remained the same; whatever his body had released was still gone. He did not need to maintain the understanding, the message, for the healing to be effective. He just needed to understand it at the time of the session. He told me, "I don't remember exactly what happened during the session, but I'm better." He understood what needed to happen to heal that particular situation, and he did it. That was the end of the story.

INDICATOR COMPASS—DETERMINING "YES" OR "NO"

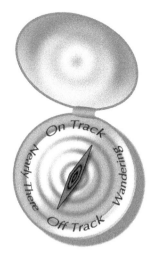

Do you know how to recognize when your client has said something of importance or made a significant connection? Do you know when she has come to an understanding rather than has more knowledge? How do you know when something important happens if she is quiet and not speaking anything aloud? Another way to put it is this: how do you know if she does not set off your "b.s. meter"?

In your given therapy, how do you know when something that your client has said, thought, felt, perceived, or done physically is significant? This is extremely important to know. It will help you keep your client on track and prevent her from leading you in circles when you have a way to determine what is significant. (There are other reasons that a client might lead you in circles, which are discussed in the section on resistance. Quite often this is when they are uncomfortable dialoguing, see chapter 6 "Dialoguing," or resistance or a protection mechanism surfaces, see chapter 11 "Meet the Twins.") I refer to the method by which you determine if something is significant as your "Indicator Compass."

CranioSacral Therapy (CST) and SomatoEmotional Release (SER) work uses a tool called a "significance detector." The significance detector is a sudden stopping of the craniosacral rhythm to indicate that something significant occurred. If you are not trained in CST/SER work, there are other ways to determine your Indicator Compass.

How do you determine what your indicator is? First, I want you to tune in to that inner part of you that is often called intuition. Second, think back to a time when you worked with a client, and she had a "Eureka!" moment. Something happened, and you were aware that something had occurred before she told you that a tension released, that she had an insight, etc. Third, ask yourself how you "knew" that something had happened. What were you aware of? The answer to this is the start of knowing your indicator. Sometimes it feels to me as if an internal compass points in the direction of "lost" or "on track" or "wandering." Once you have determined your indicator, use it to guide you as you work with clients. This Indicator Compass can help prevent you from getting dragged by your client on a wild-goose chase. Some therapists feel sensations, some see, some hear, and some are just aware.

Feel

- Something shifts under their hands.
- Something internally resonates in their body.
- The energy in the room changes.

Hear

- words or ideas
- a person's voice

See

- images
- colors
- energy move

Sense

- They have a "gut reaction."
- The energy in the room shifts or changes.

A SIGNIFICANT LACK

Your Indicator Compass can help you determine if something significant is happening. It can also indicate to you that nothing is happening. The fact that nothing is happening can be significant. It is an indication that your client needs assistance with focusing his attention on his body.

Additionally, there are situations when something should be happening in an area, but nothing is occurring. This is important information for your client. For example, your client explores his leg and notices that an area does not do what the rest of his leg does. This is important. This is an area that needs help. His body may be trying to get his attention by having nothing happen in this area. A lack or absence in an area can indicate the significance of that area.

"YOU" VERSUS "I"

While a client dialogues, he will often talk in the second person, using the word *you*. He is not talking about you, the therapist. He is talking about himself in a more indirect, more abstract nature. When used in a SomaCentric Dialoguing session, it can keep the client at a distance from the situation at hand. It can be a form of resistance, although this is uncommon. Have your client use "I" statements to help him to own the situation. Use "I" statements to help him better access the stored emotions related to the situation. Stored emotions are easier to release when he is able to recognize them. You want your client to speak using the first person ("I" statements) to have the sessions be most effective.

It is quite easy (and is sometimes humorous) to clarify what a client tells me. I will politely interrupt my client, perhaps give him a soft and gentle squeeze at a natural pause, and repeat back as a question what he has just told me. "Do you mean when *I* go for too long without eating or when *you* go for too long without eating?" Quite often, he smiles when he realizes what he has actually said about *me*. He then corrects himself and says, "When I do."

I take another moment to model for him the language he should use—"When I, Peter [his name], go for too long without eating…"—and have him repeat it using a first person "I" statement. This helps him to take responsibility for what he says and at the same time gets him back to where he was interrupted.

"THEN" VERSUS "NOW"

Similar to the use of *you* as opposed to *I*, clients will use the word *then* rather than *now*. When a client describes what happened in the past, encourage her to describe it as if she were back in the time when the event actually happened. It helps her better to be in the moment with what happened when she describes the situation in the *present* tense. Use of the word *then* allows her some distance and disconnection from the situation. Too much of a disconnect can prevent her from being fully aware of what is happening in her body.

For example, five-year-old Susie says, "Next, Mommy's boyfriend made [past tense] my brother eat the brownies; then I ran [past tense] to my room." I pause her and instruct her to speak as if she were currently there and what happens (present tense) to her. I model the use of present tense by repeating her words, "Mommy's boyfriend *makes* my brother eat the brownies, and I *run* to my room." I then have her repeat it back to me and continue the session.

If at any time you find yourself having difficulties or become ungrounded, check in with yourself about these key concepts and the session. Have you slipped away from holding the paint palette to holding the paint brush? Does your client repeat words, or does she come to an understanding of what is happening in her body? Do you follow indicators and your Indicator Compass to make sure that your client does not take you on a wild-goose chase? Do you need to bring your client back into her body by having her use "I" statements and present tense?

4 Talking Colors

In this chapter, you will begin to explore how to identify the first language and communication style that is part of the SomaCentric Dialoguing System. There are many systems that classify human personality and communication styles. Success Signals is one I have found to be very easy to learn and use. I learned about this work in a management-concepts college class the first year I worked as a full-time therapist. The surprises that can change our lives are amazing. This material changed mine in almost every way that I interacted with my clients. It helped me to understand and communicate better with my colleagues and my family.

Once you start to listen to what people say and how people think, you will begin to identify what their "color" language is. It is easy and can be quite fun. This can be infectious and begin to show up in all aspects of your life. When you are ready to learn even more, please pick up the book *Success Signals* by Rhonda Hilyer or take one of the classes her company Agreement Dynamics offers. She is the developer of this material and has done a wonderful job providing a system of identifying what language people speak. These people include your clients, colleagues, friends, family, and the grocery-store check-out clerk. When you identify their communication style, you can better understand and communicate with even the most casual acquaintance. When you speak the same color as your client, your sessions will be more effective. Your clients will start to say, "She understands me!" and "She really knows how to listen."

Similar to Myers-Briggs® or the Enneagram, Success Signals allows you to have a better understanding of how a person processes and communicates thoughts. Hilyer has identified four different styles and assigned them different "colors." None is better or more important than the others. Each person is a blend of colors, with a general tendency toward one color being dominant. When you can identify what language—or in this case what "color"—your client speaks, you can then improve your communication with him by speaking his "color" language.

A SIMPLE QUESTION?

A seemingly simple question is not always simple. To illustrate this, I would like you to pause a moment and answer the question "What did you have for breakfast?" How would you answer that question if I sat right next to you and asked you? Just go with it and not analyze what the "correct" answer might be that I want. The only correct answer is your answer to the question of "What did you have for breakfast?"

Okay, got your answer? Now, keep reading.

One day I asked my client, "What did you have for breakfast?" She proceeded to tell me the following: "Well, I went for a walk at 7 a.m., right after I got up. Then, after my walk, I came home and had to do something. Oh yeah, after my walk, I did a bit of stretching and some yoga. Then I realized that I needed to get some laundry started. So I started some laundry..."

From my perspective, she "rambled" on for two minutes until she finally answered my question: "I had a bowl of fruit and some granola—granola with yogurt."

How would you have felt spending two minutes to get a five-second answer?

Would you have enjoyed her story about her morning?

Would you have liked to know how it made her feel to have completed her exercise at the beginning of the day?

Would you have interrupted her and asked her just to answer your question?

Would you have sat on your hands and bit your lip as she kept going on?

Would you have wanted to know more about what type of fruit, and what brand of yogurt and granola, she finally ate?

Would you have inwardly or outwardly commented about how the same thing happens to you, about doing one thing, trying to get into the kitchen, but then finding yourself distracted by the laundry?

Would you have made a joke about something in her story to bring a smile to her face?

How you just answered these questions depends upon what your own "color" is and how much you would have enjoyed listening to her story. I presented this Success Signals color-language material during the first day of one of my SomaCentric Dialoguing classes. The next morning a participant told us that she had had the best phone conversation with her husband during their 30 years together. She identified that, all these years, she spoke and listened from her very "Brown" nature, and he spoke and listened from his very "Green" nature. When she was on the phone with him, she let her own Green listen to him. As such, she was much calmer and more willing to listen. He noticed the difference and even remarked on his enjoyment of their phone conversation.

Throughout the rest of this book, I will periodically refer to an aspect or nature or style of a particular "color." I invite you to revisit this chapter to refresh your memory about the different qualities of that color.

Depending upon your personality and the situation you are in, you will exhibit one or a combination of these communication styles. Most of us are combinations or blends of colors. It is helpful to identify your primary and secondary colors and the typical environments in which you exhibit these. I am primarily a Brown with Red. This comes through strong and clear at home and in circumstances when I am not working as a therapist or teacher. When I wear my therapist hat or have on my teacher's cap, I am the best Blue chameleon I can be so that I foster clear communication with my clients or students.

THE COLOR OF CLIENTS

What I mean by being the best Blue chameleon possible is that most of my clients and students want me to speak Blue to them. If they speak Blue to me, I will reciprocate. However, I always keep my ear open to be able to identify if someone is a different color, so I can speak through that filter.

When you know your own color style, it helps you understand why communication with certain people may be easy or difficult. There are natural affinities such as between Blues and Reds and between Browns and Greens. Blues and Reds are both colors that are comfortable with intuiting. Browns and Greens are comfortable analyzing. Blues and Browns are one of the more difficult combinations to communicate with each other. Blue does not care for Brown's seemingly bottom-line temperament, and Brown does not have time to hear how Blue feels about things. Reds and Greens cross paths when it comes to rules. Reds do not like rules for the sake of rules, and Greens follow them as close to the letter as possible.

When you can identify the color style of your clients, you can quickly know what language they are most comfortable speaking. Here are some real-life client examples. Try to identify each one's color. Have you ever had clients like these? How did you work with them in the past? What would you do differently now, having identified the color in which they spoke?

Have you ever had a "Molly"?

She's my client who walks into the office for her appointment. Halfway through the door, she's already "half undressed" and hops on the table. Her body language shouts, "Okay, I'm ready. Let's go!"

Or maybe you have had a "Judy"?

She comes in, sits down in the chair, and wants to know, "How was your weekend?" "What are you doing for vacation?" "How is your day going?" Before you can even begin to ask how her headaches are, you know you have to answer her questions, or else she will continue to ask you how you feel.

Then there is "Irv."

He continually inquires, "Have you heard about this new product? Will it help me?" "Do you think I should talk to my chiropractor?" "I found this information on the Internet. What do you think?" as he hands you ten pieces of paper about three different remedies for his problem.

And what about "Sarah"?

With a smile on her face, she always arrives with a good joke. She's a carefree spirit who cannot wait to tell you about her last-minute trip to the circus with her nephews.

Each one of these clients speaks to you in a different language. If you are able to recognize what their communication language is and speak their color, then you will be able to meet each one's needs more completely. You start the session quickly for Molly, the Brown, and then ask her how things are for her. You can briefly and succinctly tell Blue Judy that you had a great weekend and turn the question around back to her. You are patient with Irv as he Greenly talks on and on, wondering about all the possible things that might help him; you just treat him while he talks. And Sarah, well, all you can do is smile and laugh with her and her Redness.

So, go back to my story about asking my client, "What did you have for breakfast?" How would you have responded to her answer? If you did not enjoy her story or thought that how she felt about completing her exercise seemed irrelevant, then learning how to listen to someone who is Blue or Green could be helpful. If you easily related to her story, your own Blue is showing. If you attempted a joke, then your Red side is coming out. If you wanted more details, that is your Green nature. And if you sat on your hands, bit your tongue, or would have interrupted her, it is okay—that is typical of us Browns.

Table 1. Success Signals communication styles

Red	Blue
Intuitive more than analytical	Intuitive more than analytical
Nonlinear	Asks for input
Spontaneous	Empathizes and shares testimonials
Enthusiastic	Considers how others will be helped
"No rules"	"Hugger"
Class clown	
Green	**Brown**
Analytical more than intuitive	Analytical more than intuitive
Logical	Logical
Asks for details	Gets to the point
Linear thinkers	Wants specifics
"Tell me more"	"Just do it!"

SPEAKING THEIR COLOR

Here are some tips on how to communicate with people of other colors:

- Look over the descriptions of the different colors.

- Bring out that aspect in yourself.

- Put yourself in their shoes.

- Be intuitive-centered with Blues and Reds.

- Be fact-centered with Greens and Browns.

- Provide details for the Greens.

- Be clear and concise for Browns.

- Tell a joke or ask a Red to tell one.

- Ask how the Blue feels.

With Blues, be careful about inadvertently crossing professional boundaries. Blues like to know how you feel and your thoughts/feelings about a topic. Be careful that the conversation stays focused on your client and how he feels. It is appropriate to answer his question, which you probably get every time he comes, of "How was your weekend?" or "How are you today?" He is sincerely asking and wants to know. For a Blue, it is not just a way to be polite; rather, it is a way to connect and communicate with others.

A Red loves a good laugh, enjoys spontaneity, and does not like to fill out forms or be given rules. Again, be careful about overstepping professional boundaries with a Red client. It is easy to get joking and laughing. The next thing you know you have made a joke or unprofessional comment that was intended to be funny but was misconstrued. The best thing to do when you work with a Red is let him tell the jokes while you laugh. However, do not let that distract you from the real reason that he is in your office. Laughter can be a very good medicine and can be a good ice-breaker. It can also be a very effective mask behind which your client can hide. You may need to refocus his awareness back onto his body and to what is happening in the session.

Blues and Reds enjoy stories and analogies and anything feeling-based. You may find that these are the clients with whom you have the easiest sessions. However, if you do encounter resistance with a Blue or Red, determine the source of her resistance. If she is unsure, because she has never done this before, appeal to her feeling nature and ask her to humor you and just try it. You can give her a brief example of a session with someone else. Make sure not to reveal anything about the actual client and use lots of "Wiggle Words"—which are described in chapter 9—to express that her session may be different from the one you just described.

It takes a bit of skill to get a Green to feel what is going on in her body because she is not as feeling-centered as are Blues. Greens like to focus on facts and the logical. You may need to utilize a technique like "Mini Me" or "10 Things" or "1-2-3," described in chapter 10, "Getting Started." Bear in mind that it is likely that your Green client wants to determine what is going on logically. A Green is accustomed to figuring things out factually rather than allowing herself to feel and be aware of what is going on in her body. She has a difficult time trusting or believing that her body can communicate with her.

A Brown is similar to a Green in that she tends to be more logical and factual. While a Green will want to explore multiple options and possibilities, a Brown just wants to finish it. Browns can be impatient, so you need to keep your questions short and to the point. The best way to frustrate and alienate a Brown is to be wishy-washy with her. Be careful not to hand her ideas directly or clue her into what you notice. Wiggle Words are necessary to make a suggestion and have your Brown client own the experience.

When you encounter resistance with a Green or Brown client, determine the source of the resistance. Is it that she does not understand the process? If so, give her the facts of how a session generally works: "We're going to help you get in touch with the part of your body that is <u>holding the anger</u> or <u>causing your shoulder to hurt</u> [fill in the blanks]. It has gotten your attention for a reason. You will then talk with it to determine what it wants you to be aware of. Then, you will figure out how to resolve the situation."

Is there resistance because the client does not believe that she can talk with her body? Or does she not believe that talking will help? Suggest that she experiment and just give it a try. Appeal to her logical sense by asking her, "What do you have to lose?" She will probably quickly realize that she has nothing to lose and, possibly, something valuable to gain.

To further help overcome any resistance or struggles for a Green or Brown, it can be very helpful to utilize her audial, visual, or kinesthetic (AVK) processing language to help her become aware of what is going on in her body. To determine what her AVK processing language is, refer to chapter 5, "Frustrated Aardvarks."

Have you ever had a client with whom you dreaded talking on the phone because you knew he could talk and talk for 30 minutes without getting anywhere in the conversation? Have you ever hung up from a conversation and wondered if the person had been rude by not letting you tell him all that you thought he should know about the therapies you offer? How about the prospective client who calls a couple of times before actually making an appointment? Then there is the client whose age you wonder about because she giggles throughout the phone call.

If you pay close attention to the initial phone call from your client, you may be able to tell from that first conversation which color he is. Make a note as to your guess. When he comes in for his session, you can start off on the right foot. With your good guess as to what his Success Signals communication color is, start to talk to him in his apparent color. As your conversations proceed, if you realize he is a different color or a blend, shift with him. This way you will have him saying right from the start, "She understands me!"

Other tendencies I have noticed are the following:

- Blue has a difficult time hanging up the phone. He will say goodbye but then continue to talk.

- Red may tell you a story or a joke and be full of ideas.

- Green will keep you on the phone to inquire about all the details of your sessions. She will ask if you have had other clients similar to her and where can she find out more information. She may also tell you that she has to think about it more, now that she has some information.

- Brown just wants to know if you have an appointment available, what your fee is, and what your schedule is like. He does not care about any of the things that concern a Blue, Red, or Green. He hangs up quickly.

By now, you have a sense of what Success Signals color communicator you are. You probably have been making a mental list of some of your clients who fit into each of these categories. I have found that most therapists have a significant amount of Blue to them. As a therapist, you care and want to know how your client is—a strong Blue trait. As you have read through this chapter, you probably have realized why some clients are easier to work with than others—they speak your same color language.

For a challenging client, try to listen to her in her Success Signals color language. You may tire of repeating the same instructions to someone, but it may not be that there is a cognitive memory problem. Having to repeat things may indicate that she is Green and wants to make sure that she has all the information she needs. If you think that someone is being short and rude with you, it may just be that she is Brown and wants only minimum information. Trust that if the Brown person needs more information, she will ask you for it. If her flamboyance seems a bit too much, determine if you are listening to the dramatic nature of a Red. If so, humor her. When you understand your client's perspective, or, in this case, her Success Signals color communication style, it is easier to have patience and compassion, and the session will go more smoothly.

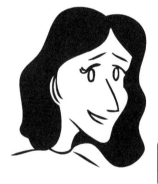

Do you need in-depth information before making a decision? *Greens* get details.

Is it important to know how others are feeling? This is a *Blue* person.

Do you like humor, freedom, to explore possibilities and fun? Go, *Red*!

Are you a bottom-line type of person? *Brown* it is.

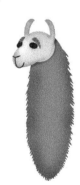

I have presented only a part of how this material can help you go beyond conversing with your client, so your client will say, "He really gets me!" There are many more ways in which this material can be applied to a variety of relationships, between individuals, between working professionals, and within organizations.

5 Frustrated Aardvarks

WHAT IS FRUSTRATED LIKE?

I want to give you a peek behind a closed door. I sit in the office of my friend—call her Dr. Milton. She is a homeopathic physician. Although I have known Dr. Milton for a couple of years, this is my first homeopathic consultation with her. I want to learn more about how she practices homeopathy.

This first consultation is generally about two-to-three hours long. A couple of my clients who have seen Dr. Milton have said that their first appointments were as long as five hours! (Two hours is a long time, and five hours can be intense.) Dr. Milton spends my session delving into all aspects of my life—my childhood, my teenage years, my relationships and marriages, my work, my goals, even my nighttime dreams.

She wants to know how I feel about different aspects of my life. How did I feel when my sister would tease me? How did I feel when my husband teased me? How did I feel when…? On and on she asks questions about how I felt in various situations. She has me free associate with different words. When I come to a particular word, she asks me "When you think about [particular word], how do you feel?" My increasingly frequent response is the word *frustrated*. So, Dr. Milton asks me "What does frustrated feel like?"

"What does frustrated feel like?" I answer exactly that—"Frustrated!"

Dr. Milton's persistent inquiry "How does that feel?" is also very frustrating. Why? Because I am the type of person, believe it or not, who has a difficult time describing what an emotion feels like in my body. If you think back to the Success Signals color descriptions, you may remember that Brown individuals are more "thinkers" than they are "feelers." I am very Brown. So, the Brown part of me that is succinct and to the point tells Dr. Milton exactly what I felt in those different situations—"frustrated." I remember a couple of times telling Dr. Milton, "There's nothing more to it than that—I just felt frustrated."

For one who gets to the point (Brown-natured), rather than someone who wades through different things (Blue or Green), two hours of this approaches torture. I sit there not even being able to imagine going around and around like this for five hours. Several times I want to say to Dr. Milton, "If you asked me the same question in a different way, rather than asking me about how it feels, I might be able to give you more information, what it seems that you are wanting." However, I do not. I (figuratively) sit on my hands and bite my lip, thinking, "She's the expert; she knows what she is doing. I am going to give her the respect that she is due and not tell her how to do her job. She doesn't tell me how to do mine, so I won't say anything." Now, maybe I should, but I do not. I am also curious as to where things will lead, and I want to observe how she handles the session.

Had Dr. Milton asked me to tell her what I *noticed* or *sensed* when I feel frustrated, she would have gotten a different response. Had she asked me to describe what *frustrated* sounded or looked like, she would have gotten different information. Unfortunately, she continued to ask me the same question repeatedly. I had a good idea about what she implied with her question. Finally, I mentally changed the question to suit my way of processing. Without saying anything to her, I asked myself the question in a slightly different way and elaborated on what "feeling frustrated" felt like. It was as if I had put a *Babel fish* (see glossary) in my ear, letting it interpret her questions into a language that I understood.

DO YOU NEED A BABEL FISH?

My first introduction to the concept of processing styles focused on how people learn. Individuals learn in a variety of ways—audially, visually, and kinesthetically (AVK). Some people are audial learners: they learn best by listening and talking. Those who are visual learners are able to understand things best when they see the material, such as words and illustrations and diagrams written on paper or on a white board. Kinesthetic learners learn most easily when they can get their tactile sense involved in the process. They learn by doing and getting their hands into or on the subject. Kinesthetic learners also learn by drawing doodles while listening or by writing and taking notes.

I began to study and observe that these processing styles also involve how people receive and communicate information. I was amazed at what started to happen with my clients when I started to dialogue with them using their processing language! We—my clients and I working together—were able to help them get in touch with what was going on in their body much more easily. We got to the source of problems much more quickly. We were able to help them work through resistance and resolve problems better. My clients did not know what had changed and what made the difference, but I did.

When I spoke my client's processing language, I more efficiently and more effectively helped him work through what previously had been perceived as stubbornness or resistance. That was not the situation at all. Seemingly, I had been talking to him in a foreign language, just as Dr. Milton had been speaking to me in a language that I did not understand. Once I had identified my client's processing language, I shifted the language that I spoke to match his. The Babel fish was now obsolete. (And that is a good thing because they were difficult to find.)

How often have you heard comments like these?

"I see what you mean."

"I feel as if I'm going to explode."

"The situation looks like this."

"If I could only put my finger on it."

"I hear you."

These and many others are phrases that are used in common everyday language. When you consciously pay attention to the situation, it is easy to interpret accurately what is meant. However, when your client is stressed or in an altered or semialtered state, he may have a difficult time reaching out for the Babel fish and correctly understanding what you mean. When you choose your words carefully, you can avoid any confusion.

When interpreted, the sentences above really mean:

"I understand what you mean."

"It seems as if I'm going to explode."

"This is what the situation is."

"If I could only figure it out."

"I know what you have said."

As a therapist assisting a client to become aware of what is going on in his body, you probably use the word *feel* quite a bit. "What do you feel?" "How does it feel?" "What does it feel like?" This is a result of lack of proper training and awareness. In the touch-therapy industry, which includes therapists such as massage therapists, physical therapists, occupational therapists, physical trainers, and movement instructors, you are taught about what the body feels like under your hands. You are taught to inquire what your client's body feels like to him in the area of concern. Have you ever said to a client, "Tell me what it feels like," but he did not know what to tell you? I am sure you have. I know I have. I really meant to ask, "What are you aware of?" From there, he could have said, "It looks like…" or "It sounds like…" or "It seems like…"

For those in the talk-therapy industry, which includes psychologists, psychiatrists, and social workers, you are used to working with emotions. You generally want to know how a situation made your client feel emotionally. This is not quite accurate. You want to determine how your client experienced the emotion or what emotions your client experienced when a situation happened. Have you ever asked your client "How did that make you feel?" and she was tongue-tied? I am sure you have. Perhaps what you really wanted to ask is "How was that for you when…?"

Regardless of the type of therapy and the reason for the session, if you ask your client "What do you feel?" he may not be able to answer. If so, it can be difficult to get information for you to help him. He may not feel anything for a few reasons:

- He does not understand the question.

- He does not know the answer.

- He does not speak that language.

What do you say? What do you do?

AVOIDING THE MERRY-GO-ROUND

As a child, I loved the merry-go-round; it was one of my favorite things to play on at the playground. I loved to run as fast as I could while I pushed it, trying to get it to go really fast. Being tall for my age, I had long arms and was a strong pusher. The other kids often said, "Push us, Julie, push us!" I would push and push and quickly run and jump on. Around and around we went! There were a few times—well, actually more than a few times—when my clumsy and not-so-coordinated feet would get in my way, and I would trip. I would fall and skin my knees and hands. Oh, how that hurt! But I would brush myself off and start all over again with the fun.

Merry-go-rounds are fun for the playground, but they are frustrating in the treatment room. When I sat in Dr. Milton's office, I felt as if I was on the merry-go-round of the playground called homeopathy consultation. Around and around we went with my trying to describe what things felt like. Had Dr. Milton known my processing language, we could have avoided the proverbial skinning of the hands and knees, the slips, and my extreme frustration for two hours.

Rather than going around and around on a merry-go-round, going nowhere fast, you want to determine if your client is an audial, visual, or kinesthetic processor. Or is she someone who simply senses? How you determine which processing language she speaks is quite easy. You simply start by asking a general question, a broadly worded question, about the situation.

"What are you aware of?"

"What do you sense?"

"Bring your attention to where my hands are. Tell me what you notice."

"Get a good sense of it. Tell me what you are aware of."

Use the words *sense*, *notice*, and *aware* where you have habitually used the words *feel*, *see*, *hear*, and *think*. I want to mention something here: please avoid the word *think*. (I discuss this more in chapter 8, "Word Choice.") You want to avoid *think* because it will bring your client into her head and start her thinking about the situation, rationalizing and analyzing it. This is what you are trying to avoid. You want to get her in touch with what is happening in her body, and if she starts to think, she brings her awareness out of her body and into her head. Avoiding the word *think* can help you stay off the merry-go-round.

To determine what processing language your client primarily speaks, use broad-meaning words in your questions. *Sense*, *notice*, and *aware* do this very well. Then, based on your client's response and her use of words indicating hearing, seeing, and feeling, you will begin to have an idea which primary processing language she speaks. Once you have an idea of this, continue to have her explore the situation using her processing language—audial, visual, or kinesthetic.

If you ever get stuck or it is difficult to find the words for a well-phrased AVK question, simply ask a broad sensing, noticing, or awareness question.

WHICH PART OF THE AARDVARK IS YOUR CLIENT?

When you open the dictionary to "A," the first illustration you generally will see is an aardvark. They are funny-looking creatures—a long snout, a long tail, big ears, no hair to speak of really—but they do look cute! They eat ants, termites, and aardvark cucumbers. Oh my! A cucumber named after them—interesting! Did you know that, according to Wikipedia, aardvarks hold a place in African folklore as animals that diligently search for food and are fearless of soldier ants?

What does an aardvark have to do with SomaCentric Dialoguing or processing languages? Well, it is an intriguing animal and word that makes me think of AVK. AardVarK. Also, when you can identify your client's processing language, you can help him more easily look for information (food) and be less afraid of what his body wants him to know (soldier ants). When you determine what specific language your client speaks, you can dialogue with him in the exact way that is comfortable for him. Imagine how unhappy the aardvark would be if you handed it a common cucumber. It would turn up its snout at you. What would happen if you handed it a Japanese cucumber? An English cucumber? Perhaps that picky aardvark would like a Persian cuke? Nope? It would be quite happy if you gave it an aardvark cucumber. It would likely give you a nice, big grin. Now it is time to learn how to determine which "cucumber" your client likes.

Audial

People who are audial or aural receive information through the sense of hearing. A sensation may be perceived through specific words, sounds, or impressions garnered from hearing something. They may learn and understand best through the act of talking and listening.

Listen to how your client talks with you. Phrases she will use in her mannerisms of speech include the following:

- I hear…
- It sounds like…
- What comes to me…
- I sense…[1]

Questions you can ask an audial client include the following:

- If it could speak, what would it say?
- What does it want to tell you?
- What does it sound like?
- Is it loud?
- Does it sound soft?
- Does it sound angry, sad, silly? (some emotion)

An audial client will be able to answer these types of questions fairly easily.

---

1   When statements include phrases such as "What comes to me" or "I sense," there may be a different processing language your client speaks. When you hear these, explore them more and listen carefully to verify her primary processing language. (Clients who are visual or kinesthetic or sensors may also use these phrases.)

Visual

Visual processors are those who receive information through images. They may see a vague mental perception. Or they may see an image as clearly as if they looked directly at it. They see, in their mind's eye, the meaning and connection of things.

Pay attention to what your client says. Phrases a visual processor will use in his manner of speech include the following:

- I see…
- It looks like…
- When I look at it,…
- It's red…
- It's big… (this can also be kinesthetic)

Questions you can ask a visual client include the following:

- What does it look like?
- If you were to look at it, what would you see?
- What color is it?
- What size is it?
- Tell me what you see.

A visual-processing client may want to show you where his body needs help. Many times a client had lifted his shirt or pant leg in an attempt to show me where his problem was, even if there was nothing remarkable to see. He just wanted me to see his leg as opposed to looking at his blue jeans.

Kinesthetic

People who are kinesthetic are those who feel—literally. To be kinesthetic means to be aware of or sense by touch or have a sensation other than by sight (visual), hearing (audial), taste, or smell. Kinesthetic sensations are perceived or sensed by touching. Kinesthetic processors understand and learn when they move or do something. They often have realizations when they experience physical sensations.

Listen to how your client talks with you. If she is kinesthetic, phrases she will use in her mannerisms of speech include the following:

- I feel…
- It feels like…
- If I touch it…

- It's hot…
- It's hard/rough/smooth… (can also indicate visual processor)

Questions you can ask a kinesthetic client include the following:

- What does it feel like?
- If you were to feel it/touch it/pick it up/hold it, what would it feel like?
- What is its texture?
- What is its temperature?
- How big is it? What is its size?

Kinesthetic processors also may put their hands (or your hands) on the area of their body that needs help. This is because they can better communicate how they feel and what they want you to know through tactile stimulation.

Your turn to start noticing

You can start to notice what type of cucumber your client wants by noticing what AVK processing language your client speaks from the time of the first conversation you have with her, whether in person or on the phone. When you sit down with her for the first time and complete your client history and intake, pay attention. What does she tell you? What phrases does she use to describe herself? What words does she use to describe her situation? It may be quite easy for you quickly to get several strong clues that reveal her style of processing.

Once your session has begun, start your inquiry with broad sensing/noticing/awareness types of questions. Listen to the answers and how the client responds. What words does your client use? If you think you have a good idea of what language he speaks, then begin to ask some questions using his language to elicit more information. Does your client readily respond? If so, keep going. If not, try a broad question again. Use his response to confirm your initial guess, and just alter your question. His response may guide you to a different AVK language.

More than one?

Does your client talk to you in more than one language? Does she talk about seeing something and later describe what it feels like? If so, *great!* It might seem confusing at first, especially if you are trying diligently to figure out what processing language she speaks; however, she is not trying to confuse you on purpose. She is probably new at this as well and not aware that she shifts from one style to another.

Actually, if your client goes from one language to another, your work is easier. If you accidentally ask a question that is not in her primary language, she will probably still be able to answer you easily.

What do I mean by "primary language"? If I say "primary language," does that imply there is a secondary and even tertiary language? Absolutely! With SomaCentric Dialoguing, you focus to ask questions and make statements using the language that your client uses most easily. This is her primary language. However, because people are dynamic and ever-changing, living beings, the language your client uses to express herself may change as the session progresses. This is actually what you want to happen.

When your client begins to articulate what is going on in her body in a variety of ways, it means that her level of awareness is deepening. As she describes further, her understanding helps peel away layers of resistance or protection, so that she is able to connect more fully with herself.

You can also actively help your client become multilingual. After you have asked your broad noticing/sensing/awareness questions and determined what her primary language is, have her describe the particular part of her body in detail using that language (AVK). Then, have her describe more aspects using another language, perhaps kinesthetic. (Switch to audial if you do not get anywhere with kinesthetic; or, vice versa, start with visual, then use audial and then kinesthetic. The order does not matter.) After a few of those questions, switch to audial. Pay attention to what happens. Your client has now started to tune into her body on a multitude of layers. Quite often, changes occur easily at this point because your client is fully dialoguing with her body. This is what SomaCentric Dialoguing's goal is—to have your client be aware of what is happening in her body at the deepest level.

Confused? Maybe the client is a sensor

Sometimes a client speaks a little of one language and a smidgen of another, with a strong flavor of vagueness. Sometimes a client does not fit into one category. I call someone who processes this way a "sensor." A sensor does not have any one language as his primary AVK processing language. Sometimes he has his eyes open and stares intently past you or up at the ceiling. He looks as if he is searching for something. He searches for that part of him in which lies the answer to your question. Sometimes he may be able to describe an awareness in general terms, and, with prompting, he can give more details. Sometimes a sensor has an elaborate story he tells that is analogous to what is happening in his body. Sometimes these stories sound nonsensical and made up, but they are meaningful to your client. Go with it. Ask him to tell you more. Have him fill in the details until he has a clear impression of what is happening with his body.

An analogy that I like to use for helping a sensor is painting a picture. Have him paint you a word picture of the situation. When you use broad questions it is as if you are giving him some pencils to sketch a rough outline. With those responses, determine if he wants to fill in with audial, visual, or kinesthetic information; this is similar to drawing with pastels, water colors, or oil paints. One style is not better than another; he just communicates the information differently depending upon his style. Continue to ask questions, using his specific language(s) to help him fill in the lines and add detail. And yes, let him mix it up. Just stay tuned in to those shifts. Continue until he has a good picture or sense of the situation.

Your own processing language

When you work with a client who has a different processing language from yours, be careful that you do not accidentally use your language instead of hers. As a therapist, it is important to be aware of your word choice when you give your client instructions. Use general terms or use her specific language. For example, if you tell your client "I am looking for you to describe what you see," she might have a difficult time if she is not a visual processor. She would understand your words better if you said, "I am wanting you to describe what you are aware of."

Use "I am wanting…" instead of "I am looking for…"

Use "I have a sense that…" instead of "I have a feeling that…"

Use passive wording when asking these questions or giving statements, rather than a more directive, active language. A more directive or active language such as "I want you to…" can be interpreted as being leading. It may also be perceived as threatening or demanding. This can bring up resistance or protection mechanisms, which make your job more difficult. Be gentle and clear, yet direct, about what you want your client to do.

PROCESSING LANGUAGE EXERCISE

How many words or phrases can you think of to indicate a client's language?

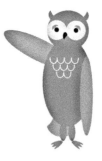

How many questions can you ask to elicit information using a client's language?

6 *Dialoguing*

You are reading this book because you want to help your clients in the most effective and most efficient manner. Perhaps you have previously dialogued with them. Perhaps a therapist has dialogued with you. Somewhere along the way, you may have discovered that dialoguing can be a useful tool.

Of course, life is always easiest when things roll smoothly. The sessions that take the least amount of effort and energy are the ones where you know what the problem is and you know what to do to help your client. The sessions that are the most cumbersome or those that drain your energy are quite often the ones where you find your techniques do not work as easily as you had previously experienced. Do you begin to wonder whether you are any good at this? If you are a bodyworker, perhaps you think maybe you should just be quiet and only do manual work. Or if you are in the talk-therapy field, you may think that you should stick to what you have done all along and not try anything new. The purpose of this book is to teach you, the therapist, how to dialogue effectively and efficiently with your clients. By the time you are done with this material, you will have a lot more information, skills, and confidence to go beyond conversing with your clients.

There are a couple of factors about stumbling blocks you might encounter. First, the problem may not be you or what you are doing. Believe it or not, it very well may be your client. I am not going to go so far as to blame your client. However, you may be doing everything "by the book," yet it may still feel as if you are pulling the rhetorical hen's teeth to get your client in touch with what is going on with her body.

Feel free to breathe a big sigh of relief and know that it might not be you. Let's explore what might be occurring. Generally, one of two situations happens.

One possibility is that your client does not want to dialogue. Yes, perhaps you have discussed with him the idea of doing something a little different or a little new. Or maybe you have not. Maybe you went with the flow, and the next thing you knew you were SomaCentric Dialoguing with him (or at least attempting to, because he showed signs that he did not want to dialogue).

The second situation may be that your client does not know how to dialogue. This chapter examines both situations and gives you guidelines about how to start a SomaCentric Dialoguing session. You will also learn about one of my favorite techniques, the Permission technique. And you will learn about when *not* to do SomaCentric Dialoguing with a client.

WHAT TO DO WHEN A CLIENT DOES NOT WANT TO DIALOGUE

Sometimes it is obvious that a client does not want to dialogue. Perhaps he has directly stated, "I do not want to do this." Or maybe he has said nothing at all, regardless of how wonderfully you have crafted your open-ended questions. Other indications that a client does not want to dialogue include his eyes glazing over (if he is looking at you), his changing the subject away from your questions, and his becoming physically restless and agitated. There are many different reasons why a client may not want to dialogue. It is now your job gently to determine and understand why he does not want to dialogue. Reasons may include that he feels unsafe, is fearful, or is afraid of being wrong or of failing. He may not want to dialogue because he does not know how to dialogue or he does not know what is expected of him. It may be something that you have said or, conversely, something you have not said.

To begin to understand why your client does not want to dialogue, ask something like "I notice that you seem to have some hesitancy about dialoguing. Is that so?"

If he is hesitant about dialoguing, the easiest way to find out why is to say, "Tell me about your hesitancy." He may straightforwardly tell you that he is not sure about what he is doing. I have had many clients get started, only to stop quickly and say, "I feel like I'm just making this up." He may tell you that he is afraid of what might come up; he may tell you something else. One can only hope that he will not deny that he does not want to dialogue. If he truly is unwilling to dialogue but denies it, then the best thing to do is encourage his willingness and try all of the following approaches.

> Understand why your client feels:
> - unsafe
> - fearful
> - fearful of being wrong/a failure
> - uncertain of what to expect
> - unsure how to _____
> - apprehensive about something you said or didn't say

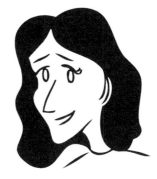

Feeling unsafe

If your client indicates that she feels unsafe, you will need to create a safe space for her. First, be present with yourself. Are you following the instruction to "*be, here, now*," as discussed in chapter 2, "Creating and Holding a Safe Space"? I hope that you are. If not, make whatever internal or external adjustments you need to make sure you energetically provide a safe and supportive environment for your client. If you cannot, accept it and use the dialoguing at a different time.

Next, find out what your client needs to feel safe. Simply ask, "What needs to happen for you to feel safe?" It is a very appropriate question that empowers her to speak about her needs. If she is unsure, ask if she needs anything in the room changed. Sometimes a client needs more or less light than there is. If there is music playing or a water fountain running, she might feel safer with different music or the water turned off. Sometimes a simple adjustment in room temperature, taking off a layer of clothes, or giving her a blanket is enough to help provide a sense of safety and comfort.

And, yes, laugh if you want, but this is true: your client may feel unsafe because she needs to empty her bladder. If this is so and you have asked the question "What needs to happen for you to feel safe?" she might tell you that she needs to use the restroom. It is amazing and wonderful how the body takes care to protect itself when it is not comfortable. A full bladder can be quite a distraction from becoming more in touch with what is occurring in other parts of her body.

Sometimes the feeling of being unsafe simply disappears once the client acknowledges her initial feeling of uncertainty. You may do something that seems minor to you, but it can make a major difference to your client. Thank your client for recognizing that she felt unsafe and for getting in touch with what she needed. I like to use this as an opportunity to educate my client about the fact that this is what SomaCentric Dialoguing is all about—listening to her body when it tries to get her attention.

Fear

You ask your client, "I notice that you seem to have some hesitancy about dialoguing. Is that so?" He may respond with, yes, he is hesitant because he is afraid of something. A wonderful way to begin a SomaCentric Dialoguing session is to explore his fear. Please do not project onto your client why you think he is fearful. Make no assumptions as to the source of the fear. You may know a lot about his past history and what is currently going on in his life, but you do not know what his fear is until he tells you. You may be able to make a very good educated guess, but it is only a guess until he tells you.

I am emphatic about this because each and every moment you try to figure out what is going on with your client, you put up obstacles and barriers to his innate inner wisdom's being willing to reveal to him and you the source of the fear. His subconscious can pick up on your subconscious thoughts and react with an attitude such as "Well, if this therapist thinks she's so great at figuring out what is wrong, then I don't need to talk at all. I'll just be quiet and lead her on a wild-goose chase." SomaCentric Dialoguing is about learning to speak the client's language and to help him be in touch with what is happening within his own body. The moment you start to guess, think you know, and act on that information, you start to move out of SomaCentric Dialoguing and into the realm of psychotherapy.

(I have just revealed one of my pet peeves! I am emphatic about certain topics because I and other therapists get tripped up by them. The fewer skinned knees and fewer therapy merry-go-round rides there are, the happier your clients will be.)

Let us refocus on fear getting in the way of dialoguing. Fears can be huge. Many clients have never been given permission to be aware of what was going on in their body. Now they are afraid to allow themselves to get in touch for fear of the unknown. Some clients were told always to suppress, deny, hide, or ignore their feelings or awarenesses. How often have you heard a client say, "When I was six my father/mother/grandma told me that I was to take care of my siblings and that there was no time for me to feel…"? There are many variations to this statement. It can be changed in a multitude of ways, all of which lead to the same result—your client is afraid to get in touch with his body's message because it is an unknown and thus inherently scary.

A fear might result from your client's having been told as a youngster that an awareness or understanding did not happen. Children have the ability to tune in with their bodies quite easily when they are given the opportunity to do so. Sometimes they are able to tune in energetically with things that are too subtle for adults to sense easily. It can be confusing—and, thus, create a fear—when someone is told over and over again that something does not exist, yet she inherently knows it does. It can be a scary or fearful situation when you ask clients to get in touch with that part of themselves that, supposedly, does not exist.

Sometimes a client will have put aside an aspect of or a feeling about himself because he never had permission to acknowledge, be aware of, and feel that part of himself. Sometimes this denial was imposed on him by another. Sometimes it was self-imposed, such as what happens during a trauma where others are involved. "I can't allow myself the opportunity to feel sad, because I have to be strong for my wife." I am sure that you can change this statement in many different ways by substituting comments of your clients. Years later, it can be unsettling for the client to be given the opportunity to acknowledge his body and that part of himself that was set aside. Your client may be afraid to feel what is held within his body for fear of revealing something scary.

For some clients, acknowledging a suppressed feeling is like cleaning out the closets when a good purge is long overdue. The anticipation about what will be found and what will have to be dealt with can be intimidating. In the long run, more time and energy are generally spent procrastinating and creating excuses for postponing than are spent actually cleaning out and reorganizing the closet. Emotions and sensations stored in the body are the same way. It is not always the proverbial situation of Pandora's box, however; I find many therapists have inhibitions about dialoguing with their clients for fear that something will come up that their clients will not be able to handle. I assert that as long as you stay grounded; maintain a safe space; ask open-ended, nonjudgmental, nonleading questions; and keep the session focused on what your client experiences in his body, you and your client will be fine. Keep referring back to the key concepts presented in chapter 3. I call them "key concepts" for this specific reason: they are concepts that are the key to a safe and effective session.

Fear of being wrong

The fear of being wrong—ah, here is when a monster tries to stick its head into your client's session. I want to introduce you to the work of Rick Carson. He is the author of *Taming Your Gremlin* and *A Master Class in Gremlin-Taming*. I have found his work with gremlins personally and professionally very helpful. Once you have read his books, I think you will too. He likes to refer to those parts that try to tell you one thing when you really know something to be different as "gremlins."

Gremlins develop from past experiences and have been with your clients since they were born. They are often a constant companion and rarely pleasant. Gremlins can be perceived as a narrator or voice in one's head. People often have more than one. I've met gremlins by the name of Judge, The Critic, Skeptic, Chastiser, and

Under Achiever, along with Goop, Icky and Black Ball, to name a few. Gremlins use your client's fears, doubts, regrets, and self-judgments against her.

Your client's gremlin wants her to see life through his eyes. He does not have her best interest in mind. It is his job to interpret and explain experiences for her; however, he purposefully misrepresents these. The gremlin uses her negative thoughts and traumatic experiences as filters to change her perception of reality. The gremlin wants his convoluted reality or twisted truths to become the client's perceptions of life. Constantly he will badger her until she believes that he is correct, when, in actuality, part of her knows this distorted truth is false.

In this case, your client does not want to dialogue because part of her, perhaps a gremlin, says that, if she tries to SomaCentric Dialogue, she will get it wrong. If she gets it wrong, she will be affirming how much of a failure she is. Without spending the rest of this book teaching you about gremlins, let me give you two suggestions about how to work with these challenges.

First, inform your client that there are no wrong answers. There is no way for her to get anything "wrong." If she pays attention to what her body wants her to know, she will be doing it fine. I try to avoid using the word *right* as that word implies that there is a wrong way to do something. But if there is no wrong way, then everything is right. You are either paying attention to your body or you are not. Just go with whatever her body tells her.

Second, I highly encourage you to pick up both of Rick Carson's gremlin books and read through them. They are enjoyable, easy reads. Once you have read one of his books, start identifying your own personal gremlins. Find out what they are about and what it takes for them to go away or, even better, to disappear. Get some first-hand experience. I have several copies of each of his books, and I lend them to clients or encourage them to get their own copies so they can learn about taming their gremlins. When a client learns about her gremlins and how to tame them, you can use her newfound knowledge to help facilitate "stuck" situations in SomaCentric Dialoguing sessions. With the material in several books—the one you are currently reading, Rick Carson's gremlin books, and Rhonda Hilyer's *Success Signals*—you have some extraordinary tools to help your clients have better sessions.

Similar to the fear of being wrong, a client may believe that she is being childish, funny, or silly talking with her body. These are highly judgmental little monster or gremlin voices in her head trying to dictate and prevent her from getting to the core of a situation. Reassure your client that she is not being silly or childish, although initially it may feel that way. I find this comes up more with people who have strong Brown and Green tendencies. When this happens, I simply say, "Give it a try. What is the worst thing that could happen?"

Generally, the worst thing that could happen is that nothing whatsoever happens; but, in all the years that I have practiced some aspect of SomaCentric

Dialoguing, I have yet to have a nothing-whatsoever-happens situation occur. My clients always leave having gained something from the session and often have finally gotten the message their bodies have been trying to communicate.

Doesn't know what is expected

This is an easy one. When a client does not want to dialogue because he does not know what is expected, simply tell him, "There are no expectations." Whatever happens in a session is what is supposed to happen. Again, encourage your client to tune in to his body. Let him know that you are there to assist and facilitate and help him when he gets stuck. And he is just to go with what happens, go with what his body shows him. Tell him there are no expected or desired outcomes or goals as long as he trusts his body.

Doesn't know how

When you ask your client about her reluctance to dialogue and she tells you that she does not know how, you can easily reassure her that you are there to help. It is your job, as the therapist, to facilitate and make it as easy as possible for the client to become aware of what message(s) her body wants to tell her. We discuss this further in this chapter.

Something you said or didn't say

If you have been reading this book from the beginning, you have learned a lot. You have also learned a lot about how speaking the right language is helpful to improve communication. In the next two chapters you will learn why word choice is extremely important.

Please pause a moment. I would like you to remember a time, during a session or a personal interaction with someone, when you said something, and your client or friend did not understand you. Think about a time when you thought you were being clear, but it turns out that communication was not as clear as it could have been. Knowing what you now know, what role did your choice of words or a difference in language styles play in the miscommunication? Take that discovery and apply it to why a client may not want to dialogue. More accurately, why is he having a difficult time dialoguing? If your client is speaking one language and you are talking to him in a different language, he may not understand. This is why word choice is important. Ultimately, this is what this book is all about. Further on, I devote an entire chapter to the importance of word choice.

You may think you have said or asked something, but your client may be having a difficulty because of what you did or did not say. Did you say or ask something in his language? If not, he can become confused or scared. To help your client (who does not want to dialogue because he does not understand what you are trying to communicate), speak his language(s). Determine what color communication style he uses and what AVK style he uses. Then, improve rapport between the two of you by using well-selected words and his style(s) of communication. Mentally review what you have said and restate if necessary. "Let me say the same thing a little differently..."

WHAT TO DO WHEN A CLIENT DOES NOT KNOW HOW TO DIALOGUE

Along with a client's not wanting to dialogue, difficulties can arise with SomaCentric Dialoguing sessions because a client does not know how to dialogue. I previously mentioned that it is your job, as the therapist, to help the client learn how to dialogue. When a client does not know how to dialogue, you need to understand why he is having difficulty. Once you know why, then you will be able to help him learn how to dialogue. There are situations when a client becomes stuck and he will need more of your help. These include when he does not know how to get in touch with what is going on in his body, when he is blocking something in his body, or when he has become disconnected from a part of himself.

Doesn't know how to get in touch with what is going on in her body

When your client does not know how to get in touch with what is going on in her body, it is your role to assist her. Ultimately this may be why she is there to work with you. At this point, it is very helpful to know her color communication and AVK processing styles. Using her communication and processing styles can help you choose words more appropriate for her.

First use the "How to Get Started" technique (as described in chapter 10, "Getting Started") to begin the process of your client's accessing what is going on in her body. You may reach a point after that where a particular objective is trying to be met, such as determining why her hip is painful but she cannot get in touch with that area. This is a good time to use some of the specific SomaCentric Dialoguing session techniques described throughout this book, in particular in chapter 10. Of particular note are the following techniques:

- Mini Me
- 1-2-3
- 10 Things
- Permission

You will find these techniques simple and easy to remember. These four techniques can be used in almost any session and at any point in the session. They can be combined and can be used as mini-stand-alone sessions.

Why your client doesn't know how to dialogue:
- doesn't know how to begin
- doesn't know how to get in touch with her body
- is blocking something
- is disconnected with part of herself
- has not been provided with the opportunity to be aware

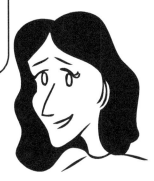

Blocking

Often, when a client does not know how to get in touch with his body, he is blocking something. This can be a form of protection or resistance and can be an integral part of his healing process. (Protection and resistance are discussed further in "Meet the Twins," chapter 11.) To synopsize, sometimes blocking can be a way that his body has configured things so that he is able to protect himself. Occasionally, this protective mechanism remains useful and needs to be honored.

However, when this protective mechanism is no longer helpful and is actually a hindrance to your client, the blockage is then referred to as "resistance." Work with resistance respectfully and gently. Often the simple act of your client's identifying what is happening in his body can help release resistance.

The best thing to do in this type of situation is help your client identify the block/protection/resistance. Determine its job or function and why it is or was there. Determine if it is still beneficial (protection) or if it is no longer necessary (resistance). If it is beneficial, a form of a helpful, protective mechanism, acknowledge it and have your client acknowledge its usefulness. And while your client is communicating with his protective mechanism, have him initiate a discussion with it. It was knocking at his door for a particular reason, trying to get his attention. Now is the time for your client to open the door and pay attention.

Protection got your client's attention; now that he is paying attention, determine what protection would like your client to be aware of. Simply have your client ask (aloud or to himself) the part of his body where the protective mechanism is, "Protection [or whatever it wants to be called], you have my attention now. What is it you would like me to be aware of?" And take it from there.

If your client determines that the block is no longer beneficial (resistance), then work with the resistance. Similar to working with protection, have your client inquire of the resistance mechanism, "What is your job? How are you supposed to be helping me?" Assist your client to inform the resistance that this type of "help" is no longer necessary (or at least not to the same degree previously). Have your client thank that part of him for all its hard work and for keeping him safe. Sometimes resistance is reluctant to leave because it does not want to die. (Yes, parts of the body take on their own personalities and concepts of living.)

In cases where resistance is still needed very minimally as a form of protection or it does not want to leave, help the client renegotiate a new job position for resistance. An analogy I like to use is renegotiating a bodyguard's job to that of a night watchman. Instead of having resistance work as a bodyguard on duty 24/7/365, exhausting to the client and the bodyguard, offer resistance a new position, a job that is less stressful, that of the night watchman. A night watchman is still able to forewarn the client about possible trouble, but he does not have to work nearly as hard as a bodyguard. This situation is easier on everyone, and everyone wins. More is discussed about "job reassignments" and bodyguard/night watchman in chapter 11, "Meet the Twins."

Becoming disconnected

Difficulty dialoguing is also about that part of your client that may have become disconnected from her conscious awareness. This may be the result of becoming disconnected from a part of herself—the physical, emotional, or spiritual part— due to a trauma she may have experienced. At some previous time, she closed herself off from part of herself because she lacked the opportunity to feel the pain at the time the situation occurred.

Both blocking and being disconnected can be tricky to identify and require sensitivity to work with. I encourage you to proceed with caution. With experience, you will feel more comfortable in situations that require your help to get your client get back in touch with the parts of herself from which she has become disconnected. Using the Permission technique, along with other methods, such as 10 Things, 1-2-3, and Guardian Angel, can help with these types of situations. (See chapter 8, "Word Choice," and chapter 10, "Getting Started.")

A form of protection that your client's subconscious may employ during a very stressful or traumatic situation arises when a part of her consciousness disconnects from part of her physical conscious awareness. Often a client will describe herself as being removed or remote from the action; she was aware of the situation but felt as if she observed it from a corner of the room. She did not feel as if she was in her physical body because the physical pain was too much to bear. It was easier for her to have her consciousness disconnect from the part of her that was in pain.

It is very important to employ careful word choice and use her communication style with this type of situation. You want to make sure that you are providing a very safe space as she begins to reencounter the part of her body from which she has been disconnected for a good period of time.

When a client has become disconnected from a part of herself because she lacked the opportunity or permission to experience the situation, sometimes the most effective and easiest way to help her reconnect with that part of her body is to give her the opportunity to feel what is going on in her body. It can be as simple as just providing the opportunity. Assist your client to place herself back in the situation. Help her become aware of as much detail as possible; refer to the "Who/what/when/where/how" section in chapter 12, "Gems and Nuances." Then, have her tune in with her entire body and pay attention to where her awareness is drawn.

When your client is aware of something going on in her body, ask her to pay attention to it and explore it. Then, using the Permission technique, give her permission to be aware fully of the part of her body from which she was previously disconnected. Giving her permission will help her become more in touch with that part of her body, and quite often she is able to reconnect, as discussed in the following example.

Meet Patricia

Patricia was about 58 years old at the time that I met her one June. She, her daughter, and I were taking a bodywork class together. During a break, she mentioned that she had a pain in her lower left quadrant and that no doctors had been able to determine the cause. She told me that every May she would get ill, occasionally deathly ill. She and her daughter were both bodyworkers and had a variety of ideas about the cause of the pain, but nothing as yet had helped, not acupuncture, Reiki, SomatoEmotional Release, or any other bodywork. Her daughter expressed great frustration and concern about her mother's well-being and indicated that not knowing the cause was difficult.

When Patricia and her daughter heard about the work I do, they wanted to know if there was anything I could figure out. We only had about ten minutes to talk about Patricia's situation. Because we only had a brief period of time, I decided to use the Permission technique, as it is very helpful when the cause of a problem has not been identified.

I led Patricia through the Permission technique and had her give herself full permission to feel fully what her lower left abdomen felt like. I encouraged her to just *notice*, just *be aware* of, just *feel* that area of her body. I did not have her say anything. I just kept her focus on her body. When she allowed herself fully to feel the pain that was there, she then realized the cause.

The insight that her body gave her amazed her. She began telling me everything that she and her daughter had previously thought it might be. Then she told her daughter and me what she had realized. Twenty years ago, while pregnant and with other little children to care for, one of her sons was kidnapped. He was then murdered. By going through the experience of giving herself permission to be aware and feel what her body was feeling, the pain, she came to the realization that she had not allowed herself to feel the loss and pain of her son's kidnapping and subsequent murder. She had not allowed herself to feel this due to her pregnancy and her other children. At that time, she consciously made the choice not to feel it because she was afraid that the negative emotions would hurt her unborn baby as well as her other children.

The messages that you tell your body can be very powerful and be carried in your tissues for years. My hope for Patricia is that her body started reconnecting and started healing from that trauma and the loss that she experienced, so that her body no longer has to react as strongly and she can begin healing completely.

WHEN SHOULD I NOT DO SOMACENTRIC DIALOGUING WITH MY CLIENT?

This is a great question. There are several situations in which you should not do SomaCentric Dialoguing with your client. There are four basic reasons not to dialogue:

- You are not comfortable with your skills.
- Your client is emotionally unstable.
- Your client is not able to dialogue, regardless of how well you and your client have tried to work through any resistance.
- Your client does not want to dialogue.

However, except for when a client is emotionally unstable, SomaCentric Dialoguing is appropriate for everyone, therapist or client.

If you are not comfortable with your skills, there are certain situations when you may want to refrain from SomaCentric Dialoguing with your client. Holding a safe space is a key concept to helping you feel comfortable. If you are uncomfortable, your client may pick up on this and feel unsafe. Sometimes beginning jitters or "gremlins" can get in the way. If you are not feeling comfortable with your skills, check your shoulder and listen in your ear. Is there a gremlin whispering to you, "Don't even bother, pal. You know you can't do it. Give it up"? If so, just get some more practice. Work with other therapists or friends or clients with whom you are comfortable. Get some sessions yourself and start talking with that gremlin. Let him know that you do know what you are doing.

One of the most important reasons not to do SomaCentric Dialoguing is a client's emotional instability. I do not recommend that you do SomaCentric Dialoguing with those who are schizophrenic, pathological liars, or have multiple personality disorder or borderline personality disorder. I would also suggest that you refer to a more experienced therapist anyone who is suicidal. And use extreme caution with those clients who have severe depression, experience severe post-traumatic stress disorder (PTSD), or are bipolar. Quite often, a client with an emotional disorder has a hard time accessing her own coping skills. If in doubt, refer out. Honor your own boundaries and limitations.

Another reason not to dialogue arises if you and your client have tried everything you know that is within his capacity, but he continues to encounter resistance or protective mechanisms. This is his body's inner knowing telling him to leave things alone at this time. Do not try to push him past his resistance. What often happens instead is that his resistance gets even stronger. "No, I'm not budging! I don't care what you learned or what you know!" "I said no, and I mean *no*!" And with that, resistance digs its heels and claws in even deeper than before.

If this occurs, just acknowledge that your client's inner knowing has other plans for the day's session and move on. Perhaps by the next session, things will have changed in some way, and your client will be more receptive and his resistance will be more willing to acknowledge what is possible.

And the most important reason not to dialogue is that your client does not want to. It is one thing for a child to say "I don't want to eat my peas" and for her mother to require that child to eat them. It is another for you, the therapist, to have your client do something he just does not want to do. Please explore the previously mentioned situations that might cause someone not to want to dialogue. At the same time, fully respect your client's wishes. Any expression of not wanting to dialogue can be a protective mechanism that you need to honor.

7 Open-Ended Questions versus Closed-Ended Questions

With dialoguing, your goal is to elicit as much information as possible, with as much detail as possible, without leading or judging the client. All of us are accustomed to asking and being asked questions as a way to obtain information. Have you ever paid attention to the types of questions a person asked when she interviewed you? The next time someone needs information listen to what types of questions are being asked.

Is the person looking for very specific information? Is she looking for specific answers? If so, it is likely that she is asking "yes or no" questions or "closed-ended" questions.

Asking a closed-ended question and not getting the desired information can be frustrating. A magazine, radio, or television interview can seem choppy or disjointed if the questions are closed-ended, creating a situation where it takes longer to get pertinent information. Asking well-constructed, open-ended questions, however, allows the person being interviewed the opportunity to communicate her message.

The next time you are in the check-out line at the grocery store, purchase a copy of one of the *People*-type magazines, a popular, general-public magazine. Find an interview or two and read them. In contrast, pick up a copy of *National Geographic* magazine or a literary journal and read some of the interviews. I think you will quickly realize that the questions in *People* are not very revealing, whereas the interviewer of the other journals has well-constructed, open-ended questions that invite the guest to reveal interesting information, to expand and explain, rather than just "yes/no" or single-worded responses.

In my SomaCentric Dialoguing classes, participants are asked to bring in an interview. We examine the questions and determine if a question is open- or closed-ended. We change closed-ended to open-ended questions. I invite you to do this on your own the next time you are reading or listening to an interview.

To get the most information during your sessions, use as many open-ended questions as possible. Closed-ended questions not only provide you with limited information, but they can also be leading in nature or imply a desired response. "You don't want to have this pain, right?" (Well, who would want pain?)

Imagine this scenario: you were in a serious accident years ago. You almost lost your life and had many broken bones. Shortly into your recovery, your orthopedic surgeon tells you that you have a choice, either to have your crushed foot amputated or to undergo multiple and extensive surgeries to save and reconstruct it. He informs you that if you have your foot amputated, you will be fitted with a prosthesis. If you have extensive surgeries, your foot will be saved, but you may have some pain for the rest of your life.

You decide that you are personally and emotionally attached to your foot. It has been a good friend and with you your entire life. And playing footsies with your loved one is very important to you. If you were to have your foot amputated, you would not be able to feel the delightful sensations of playing footsies. You decide that you would rather have some pain and play footsies as opposed to no pain and no sensations.

Now you are in your manual therapist's office receiving therapy for your foot and the pain. The pain is bearable, and strengthening your foot has gradually reduced the pain over time. Your therapist asks you about the pain, phrasing the question, "You don't want to have this pain, right?"

How does it feel having her ask you this? Are you speechless? Are you thinking, "What a huge assumption on her part"? Does she know the agonizing decision that you had to go through choosing whether to amputate your foot? Does she know that having the pain is much more desirable than not being able to play footsies? Are you thinking that your therapist may not care about you, based on her question? Does your therapist really understand you?

Alternatively, how would you feel if your therapist asked, "How is it for you having the pain in your foot?" Are you more comfortable? Do you feel that she cares and is willing to listen to you?

By asking open-ended, nonleading, nonjudgmental questions, you can easily convey to your clients that you care, that you want to hear what they have to say, and that you are willing to listen.

CLOSED-ENDED QUESTION (CEQ)

A closed-ended question is a question that is normally answered with a yes-or-no response or with specific information, often with a word or two or in a single sentence.

The question "Do you want some ice cream?" asks for either

YES or NO
a single-word answer.

With "Yes," the question was answered. The "Yes" answer tells you nothing further, such as what type of ice cream (hard, soft-serve, sorbet, sherbet) or what flavor or when the person would like it.

Hmmm, I'm not sure…

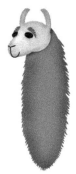

OPEN-ENDED QUESTION (OEQ)

An open-ended question[1] is one that cannot be answered with a simple yes or no or a single piece of information. When you dialogue with a client, some questions will elicit a single piece of information and may be technically considered as closed-ended questions. However, generally, it is the yes/no questions that you want to avoid. Ask questions that require your client to give you the greatest amount of information. For example, change "Do you want some ice cream?" to "How do you feel about having some ice cream?" With this question, your client can choose to tell you that he does not like ice cream but would rather have pie. This then provides you with information with which you can ask your next open-ended question to get more information and continue on with the dialogue: "Tell me more about not liking ice cream."

LEADING QUESTION

A question that suggests the answer or contains the information within it is considered a leading question, for example:

- "You'd like some ice cream, wouldn't you?"
- "You'd like some strawberry ice cream, wouldn't you?"

To avoid a leading question, you consider asking, "Is there a type of ice cream you would prefer?" However, this question is a closed-ended question, soliciting a yes-or-no answer. Even though it is not a leading question, you still want to avoid closed-ended questions.

"What type of ice cream would you like?" would be the preferred question. Even though it is typically answered with a one- or two-word answer, it is an open-ended question that allows your client to answer freely and honestly. He could even answer it with "I do not want any ice cream" if that were his preference.

Avoid leading questions because your client may feel uncomfortable answering them honestly. Many people like to please others, especially if they are a Blue person. There is also an implicit power differential that automatically occurs when your client comes to you for therapy. When you ask a leading question or loaded question (see below), your client may not want to disappoint you. He may think he will disappoint you if he gives you an answer different from what he thinks you are looking for. Open-ended questions can mitigate this power differential and your client's struggle.

---

1   For the purposes of SomaCentric Dialoguing and discussion in this book, I also consider any question that can be answered with one word but many choices as to that word to be an open-ended question.

LOADED QUESTION

Similar to a leading question, a loaded question is one that assumes that a certain situation exists and requires a yes-or-no response: "Are you still angry at your uncle?" versus "How do you feel about your uncle?" or "What are your feelings toward...?"

Please avoid these loaded questions at all costs. Initially, as you explore dialoguing, you may ask some of these loaded, leading, or closed-ended questions. This is normal and takes practice to avoid. I suggest that you practice with a fellow therapist or friend. Make a list of questions you usually ask your clients. Then, sit down with your colleague and ask a question that elicits the same or more information, by changing your usual question to one that is open-ended, nonleading, nonjudgmental, and nonloaded.

ULTIMATE QUESTIONS/STATEMENTS TO ELICIT INFORMATION

There may be many times when you feel as if you do not know what to ask or how to respond to your client. It is helpful to learn how to be a chameleon to blend in with any type of situation at any given time. I have a few choice or ultimate questions or statements that I use. They work well anywhere. Some of my favorites are:

- What are you aware of?
- Tell me what you are aware of.
- Tell me what you notice.
- Tell me more.
- What is it like?
- And...

"And..." is a good one to use when you want your client to proceed with her descriptions. It acknowledges that you have heard her and encourages her to continue.

As you will see in the next chapter, which discusses word choice, a simple way to respond to your client is to say "Interesting."

ULTIMATE QUESTION/STATEMENT EXERCISE

What open-ended questions or ultimate statements can you think of to elicit information?

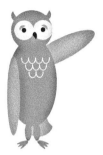

RESPONSES TO CLIENTS
Judging/judgmental responses

Just as it is important to ask the right question, it is as important for you to respond appropriately. What may seem to be benign, considerate, or encouraging may actually be judgmental. Avoid judging and giving judgmental responses. You need to recognize that, due to the power differential that exists between you as therapist and your client, your client may try to give you answers or information that results in your responding in a manner that gratifies him. You want to avoid the "Pavlov's-dog" situation.

Some examples of judging or judgmental responses that you will want to avoid include remarks such as "Great!," "Super!," and "Excellent!" Instead, use words or phrases like:

- okay
- interesting
- yup
- I understand

Occasionally, I will use "good" or "nice" to acknowledge when a client has come to a large realization:

- "That's a nice awareness."
- "You did some good work with that."

Try to limit how much you use these phrases because you do not want your client to believe that there is a correct or desired answer. There is no right or wrong answer. It is sufficient simply to acknowledge that you have heard him and leave it at that.

RESPONSES EXERCISE 1

How many words can you think of to respond appropriately to something a client has said?

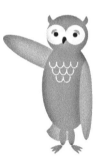

EXAMPLES OF MORE OEQS/CEQS

CEQ: Is there something your <u>stomach</u> [fill in the blank] wants to tell you? (Requires a "yes" or "no" answer)

versus

OEQ: What does your <u>stomach</u> [fill in the blank] want to tell you? ("Nothing" or "You eat too many pork rinds")

CEQ: Does it have a <u>color</u> [fill in the blank—texture, sound, feel, etc.] (Yes or no)

versus

OEQ: What <u>color</u> is it? *or* If it were to have a <u>color</u>, what <u>color</u> would it be?

Does it have a size?

Change to What size is it?

Does it talk/speak?

Change to What does it say?

Does it [fill in the blank]?

Change to What [fill in the blank] is it?

The above question ("If it were to/did have a <u>color</u> [fill in the blank], what would it be?") is helpful when a client has a difficult time because he:

- thinks too much
- believes he is making things up
- is not tuned in or aware

When a client has a difficult time, this is a great time for you to use the wonderful world of "Make Believe/Imagine/Just Pretend." Remember to avoid closed-ended questions. Ask your client to just pretend the part of his body has different aspects or characteristics to it and to answer your questions with his first impression.

Other helpful open-ended questions are ones that ask for a description of what happened with a particular situation:

What happened when you were in the <u>car accident</u> [fill in the blank]?

What happened during your <u>surgery</u> [fill in the blank]?

"BUZZER" CEQS–OEQS EXERCISE

Practice changing your questions to those that give you the most information during your dialoguing session. Let me describe to you what I do during practice sessions in my SomaCentric Dialoguing classes and individual tutoring sessions. With a group of three people, one person is the client, one is the therapist, and the third is the "buzzer." The therapist asks questions, dialoguing and eliciting information from the client. The buzzer listens attentively to what is asked. Each time a question is asked that is 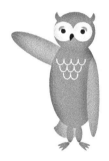 closed-ended, leading, judgmental, or loaded, the "buzzer" makes an agreed-upon sound or signal. When the signal is given, the client will not answer the question, and the therapist will ask the question in a more effective manner. When I am the "buzzer," I like to sit beside the therapist; each time an inappropriate question is asked, I gently poke the therapist with my finger and make a "buzzing" sound.

This helps the therapist recognize how many inappropriate questions she asks routinely. And the therapist can realize how easy it is to fall back on bad habits when it is difficult to think of open-ended questions or when the therapist experiences performance pressure. If the therapist has a difficult time rephrasing the question, the "buzzer" person can offer the therapist a suggestion.

STATEMENTS—GOING BEYOND QUESTIONS

Sometimes information is necessary, but you may not know exactly which question to ask in order to get the information you seek. It can be quite a frustration to know that you do not know something and do not know what information you seek. This is along the line of the saying, "I know what I know, and I don't know what I don't know." There is an easy way to discover the information from your client so the session can continue easily.

Go beyond open-ended questions. Seek the information you want by using statements. For example, your client went on vacation this summer, and you want to know about it. Start the conversation by asking, "Where did you go on vacation?" But, because you want to go beyond conversing with your client and you want to dialogue with him by eliciting information, remember to avoid closed-ended questions. A question of "Where did you go on vacation?" might get you the response of "Cuba" and nothing more. Depending upon the state of the world, politics, his job, his nationality, his family, where he traveled from, or whom he bribed, a trip to Cuba could be a very interesting story. Imagine what he might reveal if you sought information by saying to him "Tell me about your vacation."

Use a statement the next time you are at a loss or it seems there is a missing piece of pertinent information, for example "Tell me about your _____"

- pain
- accident
- injury
- headaches
- leg
- birth (when you were born)

"Tell me about your birth, when you were born." This is one of my favorites to use when I have reason to believe that a problem may be related to this time period. Sometimes I get information from my client about the emotions the client's parents experienced when the client was in utero. Sometimes he remembers something else through a stream-of-consciousness thought. "Well, I don't remember Mom saying anything about my birth as being unusual." Pause, pause, pause. "Oh yeah, when she brought me home, my brother dropped me on my head. I had forgotten that." It is amazing what clients seemingly forget or do not know can be important.

And sometimes what is remembered can be a revealing emotional connection. "Well…, when I was born my mom was sick and wasn't able to take care of me. She had gained a lot of weight and didn't know how to nurture me. I would wake up and start crying anytime someone tried to put me down for a nap or bed."

Another example is to say to the client, "Tell me what happened _____"

- to your neck
- after your surgery

Your inviting statement can open a huge door and reveal some profound information. Have your client give you a narrative, when he gives you seemingly disconnected bits and pieces of information. Pay attention to your Indicator Compass to get a clue into the pertinent piece of information that can take your client deeper into dialoguing with his body:

"Tell me what happened to your wrist."

"Then what happened?"

"Tell me about the wrist surgery."

"What were you aware of?"

RELATING STATEMENTS TO COLOR PERSONALITIES

When you say "Tell me...," you are being directive. Up to now, the discussion has been about asking and inviting your client to tell you information. Sometimes statements or directions are necessary, such as when you tell your client to climb on to the massage table or to have a seat, or that her session is over. These comments are customary and expected. When you tell someone something of this nature, it helps frame what is expected of her and helps put her at ease if she is not sure what to do.

However, when you give her a statement such as "Tell me about your surgery" and the subject is emotionally sensitive, it may be uncomfortable for her to comply. You can avoid discomfort if you pay attention to the person's Success Signals color (see chapter 4, "Talking Colors," for a review) and to how you present the statement. In general, when told to do something, a Blue will oblige because she wants to please you. Reds do not like rules, but if you ask her to tell you a story about the situation in question, she will oblige since she likes to tell stories. For the Blue or Red person, if the statement is too sharp, harsh in tone, or too quick in delivery, it could be perceived as bossy and make her feel uncomfortable. When you give a statement to such a client, be sure to bring forth your own Blue or Red nature to soften the directions.

Browns will accommodate because they like to be told what to do. Browns like directive statements as they prefer to get to the point.

Be cautious, however, when you elicit information from a Green with a broad statement. She may give you much more information than you wanted or needed. You may need to keep an eye on the session clock, as a Green will give you lots of details and background information. Some of this information may wind up being pertinent, so be sure not to tune it out. If necessary, gently steer your Green client back on track by restating your statement with a little more specificity—"Tell me about the day you broke your leg"—rather than the original statement of "Tell me about when you broke your leg." The revised statement gets you to a particular time period, whereas the original statement could also provide information about errands she ran that day, the first time she broke her leg, or the shoe salesman who told her a horror story about when he broke his hand. Some of the information with the original statement, such as the first time she broke her leg, may reveal a stress pattern held in her body or a continuing emotional fear. However, the salesman story or list of errands may not be very revealing.

Your Green client may seem to wander in his narrative response to your statement. Remember, you seek information which you can use to help solve problems. Pay attention to your Indicator Compass.

When you soften a statement, be cautious about accidentally turning it back into a closed-ended or yes/no question. It is easy to go from "Tell me about your injury" to "Will you tell me about your injury?" Avoid "Will you…" and "Can you…" as these will turn statements into questions. A simple way to soften a statement is to start with the magic word—*please*. "Please tell me about your injury." As our parents taught us, the word *please* can work magic. And, of course, if you are halfway through your statement and you realize that you forgot to say "please" in the beginning you can always end the statement with "please": "Tell me about your accident, please."

Another way to soften a statement is to say it with a smile. A wonderful way to change your tone and energy is to speak with a smile. Even if your client does not look at you and cannot see your smile, it will come through in your voice, making her more comfortable to comply with your statement or direction.

When you use statements, listen carefully to the response you get from your client. Pay attention to whether she is dictating an analytical or a logical story from memory and not present in her body or if she is able to respond with a body-centered awareness. If she mindlessly reiterates a story, help direct her back into her body. Rephrase the statement by directing her "little girl Sally" to answer or have her leg tell you what happened. This type of direction can help take her out of her brain and back into her body-awareness.

CEQS TO OEQS INTERVIEW EXERCISE

Find an interview from a magazine, newspaper, or Web site. The interview must be in the format where the question is written out and then the response is written out. It can be on any subject matter. Choose a source that is written for the general public. A good place to find these interviews is in the magazines by the grocery check-out stand (for example, *People, The Examiner, Red Book*, etc.).

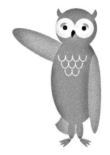

For example, look for an interview that reads like this:

Q: Is it hard work being a ballerina?

A: Yes.

Q: You have done 38 productions of the *Nutcracker Suite*. I'm sure you're tired of it, aren't you?

A: Actually...

Now read through the interview. Identify which questions are closed-ended and which are open-ended. Change the closed-ended to open-ended questions that would elicit more information. If you come across a question that is leading or judgmental, change the question so that it is open-ended and not leading or judgmental.

---

20 QS EXERCISE

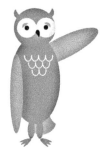 Find a couple of friends or colleagues to do this exercise with. Although the game "Twenty Questions" is done with yes-or-no closed-ended questions, this exercise uses open-ended questions. The intent is to practice dialoguing and to ask questions that elicit information. Determine the length of time during which questions are asked, for example 20 minutes. One person acts as the client and chooses a subject to tell a story to the other person, the therapist. The therapist asks questions or makes statements to elicit information. The subject or story can be real or fictitious—for example, a new job, a cat gone crazy, or a wild and wacky vacation.

Use open-ended questions or statements such as "Tell me about your vacation," "Tell me more," and "How did you feel about it?" With these, the therapist elicits as much information as possible in the specified period of time. If you run out of questions before time is up, review what has been told and try to find a tangential subject about which to ask more questions to gather more information. Continue until time is up.

8 *Word Choice*

What your client says is important. Are you aware that what you say might be even more important? It is true. What you say can shape how your client responds to you. What you ask or say to a client and how you do so determine what he tells you. This chapter explores the importance of what to say and what not to say, so that you can help your client get in touch with what is going on in his body more effectively.

Sometimes a client only tells you what he believes you want to hear. This is indicative of a Blue Success Signals color communicator. Sometimes a client will answer the very specific question that you asked, not reading further into your question. This might very well be a Brown person. And sometimes he tells you what you are implying you want to know. Or, especially if he is Green-natured, he will ask you what you mean. The best way to make it easiest on everyone is to be mindful and specific with your word choice.

In this chapter, you will learn why choosing your words is so important. The concepts that you will learn include using positive rather than negative words, emphasizing feeling as opposed to thinking, avoiding what might be construed as judgmental responses, and using humor appropriately. There are certain words that you should avoid using: *pain, problems, relax, safe*. When you avoid using these words, your clients can communicate more clearly with you. And there are questions that you are better off rephrasing, for example: "How are you?" "Is there anything that I should know about?" "How do you feel?"

NEGATIVE VERSUS POSITIVE

I can tell you, "Choose words that do not have a negative connotation." Or I could say, "Choose words that have a positive or neutral connotation." The double negative in the first sentence can be confusing, so let me rephrase: Avoiding negative words can help eliminate any misunderstanding. By saying, "Choose positive or neutral words," I am being clear and specific. You immediately know what I am communicating. When your client is in the middle of a session, she may not be very articulate and lucid, so it is important that you be clear, specific, and to the point.

At a seminar, I overheard part of a conversation. One of the participants was talking about his health concern and mentioned that he had had testicular cancer twice. (He seemed to be young, late 30s or early 40s, and relatively healthy.) The person he was talking with immediately responded with "Bummer!" He assumed that the man had suffered something undesirable by having to go through cancer twice.

The first speaker's response to the "Bummer!" comment was "Actually, it was great!" I did not have the opportunity to hear his reasoning, but he went on to explain why it was a great experience.

I mention this story because you, the therapist, may perceive something as a negative situation, yet it may actually be helpful to your client. What to you seems negative may be a learning experience or a form of protection or protective mechanism for your client. Before you respond to a client with words with negative connotations, find out how the experience was for her. It can also provide you with a lot of useful information for her session.

BEING NONJUDGMENTAL

Often your client wants to please you. This is especially true of a client who has a Blue Success Signals nature. If I had a nickel for every client who told me he did the self-care homework that I gave him, especially a couple of days before a session, I would be able to retire. Well, maybe not that many clients. My point is that when a client thinks about his upcoming session, quite often he thinks to himself, "I have my appointment with Julie in two days. I better make sure that I do my homework so she can be proud of me." If you are like me, you want your client to do his self-care homework to take care of himself, not to please you. Even though this is a part of human nature, you want to avoid reinforcing his desire to please you, his therapist.

I inquire about homework at each session. I thank my client for being honest with me when he tells me he forgot to do it, got busy, or lost his directions and therefore could not do his homework. I need to remain nonjudgmental. I explain that I would much rather have him be truthful than try to please me. I explain that now I have information about why he might not be making the progress I expect. I am not as befuddled when he is honest and tells me he did not do his homework.

I encourage the client to do his homework without chastising him. If he is not doing his self-care, then I inquire about what needs to happen for him to do his homework. Quite often, it is something as simple as just taking the time to do it. During this conversation, I try to keep my tone of voice relaxed and neutral and to remain nonjudgmental in my attitude. If I am judgmental about his not doing his homework, it comes through in my voice. It is his choice; the consequences are his as well.

How you respond to and acknowledge what a client says during a session is extremely important. You want to make sure you use words or phrases that are nonjudgmental. If you say, "That's good," you are making a judgment about what just occurred—your client just said or did something that was positive or beneficial. Society's customary reaction is to give a positive action some positive feedback. Think of Pavlov's dogs.

You want to avoid making "That's good" type of statements so you are able to remain nonjudgmental. You want to avoid saying anything that encourages a client to give you a response that elicits your positive feedback and that discourages her from giving a truthful response.

"That's interesting" is my favorite phrase to use instead of "That's good." You can easily use this statement when you do not want to make a judgment but think that you need to acknowledge what your client has said. Acknowledging what your client has said indicates that she has been listened to and heard.

When you do not know what to say, you can use "Interesting." Other comments I use include "Hmmmm" or "Uh huh." "Tell me more" is a great phrase to encourage your client to examine the situation further and provide you with more details and information. "Keep going" encourages her to continue what she is doing, indicating she is on track without actually giving approval.

In the previous chapter, we explored the concepts of using nonleading and open-ended statements and questions. Those concepts, combined with a nonjudgmental attitude, help your sessions remain neutral. This helps your client and you to remain in a grounded state and helps provide an environment of feeling safe to explore what her body wants to tell her.

RESPONSES EXERCISE 2

How many words can you think of that are nonjudgmental, which can be used as an appropriate response to something your client has said?

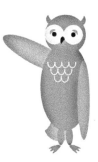

NO-NO WORDS

What do I mean that you cannot say certain things? Well, the truth is you can say anything you want to your client, but if you want to help your client most effectively to get in touch with what is happening within her body, there are words that are best avoided—"no-no" words. These include the words *relax, pain, problems, stress, think,* and *safe.*

I encourage therapists of all varieties to avoid using these words. While most of my examples are based on manual, hands-on therapies, these same concepts apply to a talk therapist or non-hands-on therapist. Therapists of any sort should avoid using No-No Words. Your client, however, is welcome to use them. It is appropriate if a client uses a No-No Word. There is no need to educate your client about such words or to have her avoid using them. You, the therapist, want to avoid using No-No Words because it can lead to ambiguity and mixed messages that work against you and slow down the session. Let's examine each word in detail.

Relax

How many times have you picked up your client's arm or leg and felt tension in it? If you asked him to tell you when he was relaxed, you might get a quick reply of "Well, I am right now." But under your hands, you can feel the tightness and heaviness of his muscles. He probably thinks he is relaxed just because he is in your office. Or just because he is not working, your client thinks he is relaxed. Or just because he is breathing, he thinks he is relaxed. The word *relax* is a No-No Word because it is not very effective in helping your client to achieve the desired state of relaxation.

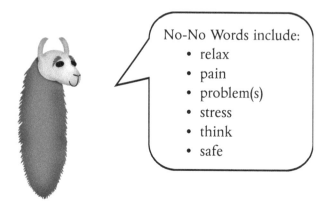

No-No Words include:
- relax
- pain
- problem(s)
- stress
- think
- safe

Have you ever lain on your chiropractor's table and, just prior to adjusting your neck or other painful area, he tells you, "Now just relax"? When I am on the chiropractor's table, I am often being twisted and turned into positions that make me feel like pretzel dough. Then when he has just the right twist, my muscles are past their comfort zone, my uncomfortable nerves are screaming to my brain, and I am feeling every kink, I hear "Now just relax" right before the adjustment as he puts my bones back in place. Does he really expect me to relax?

I am one of the millions of people who benefit from regular chiropractic care. I have booked a lot of table time with many chiropractors. There should be revolving doors going into a chiropractor's office. There is always someone coming out as I go in and someone coming in as I go out. I think you know what I mean. Imagine this scenario the next time you get an adjustment from your local friendly chiropractor. Just as he has you in your pretzel twist, he says to you, "I want you just to soften your neck." That changes the whole energy of the situation. Your body says, "Oh, he wants me to make my neck soft. Soft feels squishy, pliable, loose. Soft means to not be hard or rigid. We can do that. Let's do it for him."

Instead of *relax* use
- soften
- melt
- unwind
- let go

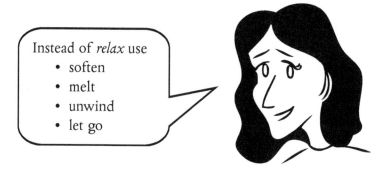

Bodies love to be helpful. You, as a therapist, just need to avoid using trite phrases that have lost their meaning. "Just relax" is one of them. Also consider that there may be negative connotations that a person may associate with the phrase. He may have been told over and over again by a nagging spouse or relative "Just relax! There's nothing to get bent out of shape about." Your client's body can get awfully confused. First, he has negative associations with being told to "relax." And then he is told to relax when he is on the chiropractor's table or your massage table, and then thinks he is relaxed. What is your client's body to think and do? It could do more if you gave him a different message.

Think about it.

What does it mean to relax? When you think about the physical state of your or your client's body, you quickly realize that there is a particular feel to it.

RELAX SYNONYMS EXERCISE

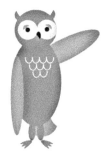

How many words can you think of to describe a state of relaxation?

Pain

I am going to be very honest with you. Using the word *pain* is a pet peeve of mine. If you read the introduction to this book, you understand why pain is a No-No Word.

Picture this scenario: your client comes in complaining that her shoulder hurts. You ask her where her pain is. She hesitates as she considers how she is going to answer your question. She hesitates because she does not really consider herself to be in pain, just that her shoulder hurts. Her subconscious is thinking, "She doesn't understand me. I told her that I hurt, not that I am in pain. Doesn't she know that pain and hurting are different?"

"My shoulder hurts" is not equivalent to "My shoulder is painful." Sometimes there will be an awareness of something hurting or being prickly, hot, cold, stabbing, achy, burning, cramping, etc. However, it is not always pain that is experienced. Often these descriptions are automatically associated with the word *pain*.

When you ask your client "Tell me about your painful shoulder" or "Where is your pain?" she may not be able to answer simply because she does not have pain. SomaCentric Dialoguing is all about effectively communicating and building rapport with your client and helping your client get in touch with what is going on in her body. If you equate the words *hurt* or *sore* or *stiff* with the word *pain*, you are working against yourself.

Discomfort is a good general term to use, instead of using *pain*. It is broad enough to cover anything from a minor ache or soreness to something extremely unpleasant.

When your client is fully alert and oriented, she can clarify: "Well it's not pain that I feel. It's actually [fill in the blank]." To expect your client, who may be in an altered state during the session, to clarify that she is not feeling a pain requires her to come up into her head (creating a thinking process) and out of her body. Often it is not desirable to bring her out of her body-awareness into a thinking process. You want to choose your words carefully.

Stick with the word *discomfort* or one similar, and you will go far.

PAIN SYNONYMS EXERCISE

How many words can you think of that a person might use, instead of the word *pain*?

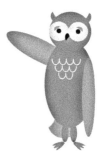

Problems

Is something a problem?

Is something a problem if you perceive it to be so, but your client has learned to accommodate it?

Is something a problem if you perceive it to be, but your client learned a valuable lesson from it?

Problem is a No-No Word. Just because you perceive something to be a problem does not mean that your client believes his situation is a problem. In the beginning of this chapter, I mentioned someone having twice had testicular cancer. Was that a problem for him? Well, maybe it initially caused many changes in his life. However, he was glad for the experience. His unconscious would have to start correcting you and justify why his cancer was not a problem if you happened to start talking to him about his cancer as if it was a problem.

The term *problem* can also arouse strong negative feelings for a person. He may be in denial that there is actually a problem. He may not want to face the "problem." *Trauma* is similar and has even stronger negative connotations for people. Find out what your client's situation is before you start considering it a problem and referring to it as such. If he uses the term *problem*, then it is very likely that he is considering his situation to be such. If he does think there is a problem, here is a wonderful opportunity to help him think positively about the situation. Use a word that does not have a negative connotation. Other words to use are *concern*, *discomfort*, or *situation*.

Words such as *concern*, *discomfort*, or *situation* do not have the societal, negative connotations associated with words like *problem* or *trauma*. I like *situation* because it allows my client to expand upon what he is telling me. When I say, "Tell me about your problem," he will often focus on the area of complaint and limit what he tells me to his aches and pains and their duration. When I say, "Tell me about your situation," he interprets this statement more broadly. Often he will tell me about how something happened, how he felt at that time, and what else was going on in his life. And he will also tell me about his aches and pains. The additional information is very helpful. It provides avenues that invite me to help him explore possible connections between what was going on in his life and his "problem."

The word *injury* is another term that I try to avoid using. It limits your client's focus to just what is bothering him. And it may not have been an injury; it may be something that has been building up over a period of time. If it is an actual injury, I acknowledge it as such and then broaden how I refer to it so that I can gather more information.

Below are good words to use:

- discomfort
- concern
- situation
- experience

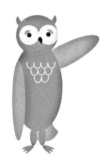

PROBLEM SYNONYMS EXERCISE

How many words can you think of instead of the word *problem*?

Stress

Similar to the words *pain* and *relax*, *stress* can be described in many different ways. One person's stress may not be the cause of stress for another. If your client appears to be stressed, do not assume it is so. Ask her what is going on. Use lots of Wiggle Words if you need to use the word *stress*. If your client uses the word *stress*, ask her to clarify what she means so that you understand her accurately. Once she has defined what her stress is or how she experiences it, find a word or phrase that she has used. Use this as an alternative to using the word *stress* when you are talking or dialoguing about her stress.

For example, your client may be wound up and overworked. Your client may be tired. Your client may be mentally overloaded. Each of these is a different type of stress and has a different cause. Even though stress is the root cause of all problems, it is a broad and unspecific word, hence a No-No Word. To keep communication clear with your clients and your dialoguing most effective, avoid using the word *stress*.

STRESS SYNONYMS EXERCISE

How many words can you think of instead of the word *stress*?

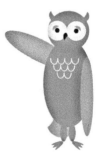

"Feel" versus "think"

I described feeling versus thinking in chapter 5, "Frustrated Aardvarks." Here I elaborate further on why it is important to be careful of your word choice when using the words *feel* and *think*.

Imagine during some wonderful SomaCentric Dialoguing that your client has a realization. You find yourself asking, "So, what do you think about that?" And with your client's answer, the session grinds to a snail's pace. What happened? Well, you just asked a question that requires your client to interpret whatever he realized. When you or your client use the word *think*, it brings him into his head and out of his body-awarenesses.

Interpreting is something for the psychotherapists to do. As a manual therapist, I do not interpret anything for my clients. And I do not want my client interpreting anything either. When you ask your client to "think" about something, it interrupts his body-centered awareness process. It easily gets his left-brain, logical part working. It interrupts and impedes the messages that your client's body wants to communicate. When you ask your client what he "thinks" about something, it keeps him in his head. Encouraging your client to "think" can help him avoid the process of tuning in, becoming aware, and noticing what is going on in his body.

Having your client "think" about something brings him up into his brain. Brain knows a lot, or so it thinks. Body knows a lot, often a lot more than what it is given credit for knowing. And Body is often not listened to enough. Please do not encourage Brain to take over. Body has been ignored and not given enough attention. It is now Body's turn to do the dialoguing.

And I have found that those who are Brown or Green communicators tend to be more comfortable as thinkers rather than feelers, so this applies to them even more.

If you have identified that your client is a kinesthetic processor or perceives awarenesses primarily through feeling, then you can use the question "What does that feel like?" But until you know your client's AVK language, ask, "What are you aware of?" or "What do you notice?" or "Tell me more." These cover all the processing language bases—see/hear/feel.

You can also ask, "Where does your awareness take you?" I try not to limit my question to a specific part of the client's body since his awareness might need to take him to an emotion rather than a physical part of his body. He might need to explore the sadness he feels that may be held in a general, nonanatomically descript area of his body. However, if you need to have your client focus on a specific part of his body, you can ask, "What part of your body are you aware of?" This helps him to narrow his awareness to a part of his body, rather than identify an emotion.

THINK SYNONYMS EXERCISE

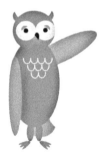

Think of other questions instead of "What do you think?"

Safe

Humans are hardwired, programmed to protect themselves and others in moments of danger. The moment that your client starts to shed a tear, cry, looks scared, or even terrified, your instincts kick in, and you have a natural reaction to reassure her that she is safe.

"It's okay; you're safe."

"It's safe now."

These are phrases that most of us have heard from our mothers at some point in our lives. They are words of soothing and comfort. Sometimes a hug or a sweet, soft, and healing kiss accompanied them. They were appropriate when there was a nightmare or a skinned knee. They are *not* appropriate for therapists to give. In the treatment room, a tear or frightened look is an entirely different situation from what it is on the playground.

Safe is a No-No Word. Phrases that include the word *safe* are to be avoided. If a client is experiencing emotions or pain associated with a past trauma or situation, she may not feel safe. It can be counterproductive to tell her that she is safe when she is, in fact, not feeling that way. SomaCentric Dialoguing is about helping your client get in touch with what is going on in her body. This specifically includes being in touch with feelings of not feeling safe. It is an important landmark when a client is able to identify that she does not feel safe. When she makes you aware that she does not feel safe, you have been given a lot of information with which you can begin to work.

We are therapists because we want to help others. We want them to be able to have a healthier and more enjoyable life. If your client indicates that she does not feel safe, it can sometimes trigger something in you that wants you to take care of her. Do not rush to do this. You need to check your boundaries as well as make sure that you are grounded. Reflect on your motivation as to why you are feeling that you want to make your client feel safe. (If you find this happening,

---

I suggest you read Nina McIntosh's *The Educated Heart*, which has wonderful material about healthy boundaries. In addition, Suzanne Scurlock-Durana teaches about boundaries and grounding in her "Healing from the Core" workshops and in her book *Full Body Presence*. More information is in the resources section of this book.)

Once you have confirmed that you are grounded and centered, what do you do? An alternative to telling the client that she is safe is to have her check in with her body and have her find out if she is safe. Having your client determine whether she is safe places the power in your client's hands. It helps her get in touch with what is going on in her body. Maybe the tear was actually one of relief, a simple release, with no emotion connected with it. Maybe her strange look indicated she did not understand something you said. The look may have been a memory flashing in front of her and, now it is gone, nothing for her to be concerned about.

What if the reexperience/awareness she is having does not feel safe? What if she feels she will not be okay? Again, this is the beginning of uncovering extremely useful information. If your client has an awareness that she is not safe, have her describe the situation to you. Help her become aware of the situation and have her figure out what it is that she needs. Then, using any tools that you already have and what you are learning here, assist her with what she and her body need to have happen.

I want to take this opportunity to introduce a technique that I like to call the "Guardian Angel." This technique is wonderful to use when a client needs assistance in accessing a past situation, especially one in which she did not feel loved, safe, or protected. The past situation may have been one where she had been abused or assaulted, emotionally, physically, or sexually. You can use this technique at any point. It helps to bring about awarenesses, realizations, and, sometimes, creative solutions. The Guardian Angel technique has a basic format that can be adjusted for each client's particular circumstance.

GUARDIAN ANGEL TECHNIQUE

You client is in a situation where she has expressed she does not feel safe (interpret this broadly).

1. Have your client get a good awareness of the situation.

2. Have her, if she is willing, describe the situation to you out loud. Having her tell you about it helps to deepen her awareness and keeps her from drifting off.

3. Have her describe to you how she is feeling, what emotions are connected to the situation.

4. Have her find out (from her body part, her little child, her inner child) what she needs to feel safe, protected, and secure.

Quite often she will need someone (real or imagined, living or passed on) to hold her, tell the offender something, or make the offender go away. Sometimes she needs someone to reassure her that she is loved, cared for, bright and intelligent, smart, wanted, etc.

5. Have her invite that person or being to be there with her.

Occasionally, this person is the client's adult self, who has learned a lot about life and has wonderful words of wisdom and the benefit of hindsight.

6. Invite the person to give your client any information or message that would be helpful for the given situation.

7. Have your client make sure that the part of her that is being spoken with and comforted really understands the message that she is being given.

This is similar to the Permission technique. Sometimes the client will know intellectually what is being said to her, but it takes some time to sink in and absorb what is being communicated so that her body understands it.

An example

Susan is in her 50s. The intention for her session was to explore her not being able to express herself fully and comfortably. She explained to me that even when she is with family and friends, she has a difficult time feeling safe saying what she wants. She explained that she always sounds unsure and has difficulty articulating what she wants to express.

We—Susan and I, working together—had her explore the situation and go back to the first time she remembered feeling that way. Initially, she found herself in fifth grade. She started elaborating a bit and then realized, "No, it was earlier than that—it was third grade. I thought I had worked this out, but I guess I haven't."

I said, "I want you to get a good sense of that third-grader. What is her name?" Susan answered, "Susie."

She got a good sense of Susie and described the situation. It was "Show and Tell" day. That day she was going to tell about her heritage. She went to the front of the class and wrote her full name, first and last, on the board. Then, in a perfect Spanish accent, she pronounced her full name. Before she could explain to her class that her parents were from Spain, the class burst into laughter. She was utterly confused. She did not know why the kids were laughing at her. She did not understand why the teacher was not doing anything. She felt so miserable. She hung her head and slowly walked back to her desk. She tried to blink back the tears. All the while, the kids were laughing, and a part of her was telling her, "See what you did—you tried to say something and it came out wrong. You're not going to speak your voice anymore if it means this type of treatment."

While Susan was on the table describing this event, her hands got ice cold, and she started experiencing the anxiety that often came when she would speak.

We had Susan give herself permission to feel all the feelings that third-grader, Susie, was feeling. As Susie was describing what was going on, I had a sense that adult Susan would probably be Susie's best resource, as her guardian angel. This knowing on my part comes from experience. Sometimes there is a sense that your client might need the teacher in this situation or parent to help. (If none of these people could be a resource for her, then I would have asked Susie directly who could help her.)

Then, I asked adult Susan, "What would you like third-grade Susie to know?"

Adult Susan gave Susie a hug and told her that she was brave for going up and doing what she did, that she had a beautiful name and a beautiful voice. Susan told Susie that it was okay to use her voice and not to give away her power to the other kids by not speaking.

We asked Susie if there was anything she wanted to ask Susan as her guardian angel. Susie asked, "Why didn't the teacher do anything? Why did the kids laugh at me?"

We then had Susie ask the teacher directly: "Go ahead and ask her." Having Susie ask the teacher directly gave her power, rather than relying on me as the therapist to rephrase the question to the teacher.

Once Susie asked the teacher and the teacher answered, there was a dramatic change in Susan's body. She was softer, her heart was not racing, and her hands were warm.

We made sure that Susie fully understood and felt what Susan and the teacher were telling her before we went further.

With the last part of the technique, toward the end of this session, we had third-grade Susie bring forward the feelings and new understanding into her life. She brought it forward through her elementary-school years, middle school, high school, into her 20s, and all the way forward to the current day.

I said, "When you get to the current day, just let me know." Susan opened her eyes eventually, then said with a huge smile, "Thank you."

This is one variation of the Guardian Angel technique. The premise is that the client is in a position of vulnerability and her guardian angel helps by providing information or intervention. In this example, adult Susan could have spoken with the teacher and the students if that was what Susie needed. In other sessions, clients have a grandparent come and look after them or have a parent or other relative tell the parent how to treat the client. Sometimes the client is not a child in the session but an adult who needs someone (real or imagined, living or passed on) to help her with a more recent or current situation. It is a wonderful technique to use when a client needs resolution of a situation when she did not feel safe.

MORE ABOUT THE WORD "SAFE"

Imagine this scenario: Your client is remembering back to a time when he was only days old. He has an intense and doomed feeling that he and his twin are not wanted. They have no crib, so they are kept in the top drawer of a dresser. He has a memory that he feels as if he is about to be flushed down the toilet. He describes that he is afraid to die, to be flushed down the toilet. He also describes that he wants to die because not being loved and not being wanted is too painful to bear.

He does not feel safe. There is no one to help him by being his guardian angel. Words are not going to soothe this over for him. His feeling of going to be flushed down the toilet may have been the perception of an infant who does not know what is happening around him. These feelings may have been real. Either way, the client experienced them as if they were real and that is what was important—his perception and experience.

This was not the first time I had experienced a client who previously wanted to die. The first time it occurred was scary for me as the therapist. I remember thinking to myself, "Oh, my goodness! What do I do? I've never been taught what to do in a situation like this. Oh, no, she can't die!" Then, my training and rational brain kicked in as I grounded myself. My client was living and breathing in front of me. She was alive. My client did not die. Something happened along the way that allowed her to live. But I did not know what it was. My client did know, though. "What would happen if we gave her permission to just be with that feeling?"

So that is what we did. We used the Permission technique. We gave her permission to feel all those scary feelings. In her situation, she was so young and tiny and vulnerable that it was too frightening for her as an infant to allow herself to feel those feelings. Part of her had disassociated with herself in order to survive.

Your client may at one time, when feeling unsafe, have disassociated from his body. He may have consciously or unconsciously disconnected some part of himself from his body. Quite often when a client is describing what is happening, he will say something like "I left my body" or "I am looking at myself." These are indications that the part of him that is responsible for keeping him safe did so by removing part of him from his physical body. This is a typical protective mechanism.

Telling your client in the most reassuring manner that he is safe and okay will do nothing to help him understand that he is safe. Part of your client is not connected to the rest of his body. For him to reconnect, he may need the safe environment of the session room to be able to feel the discomfort. Give him permission, using the Permission technique, to feel the discomfort and fear and any other emotions that might arise. He needs to have his body be able to feel and express what it needs to be able to reconnect with his disassociated part so that healing can occur.

Back to my client, the infant who wanted to die. I held a very safe space for him. We gave him permission to feel all those things that he felt. We gave his body permission to feel them. While we held a safe space, I constantly checked in with myself to make sure that I stayed grounded. Once his body was able to experience the situation fully, not disassociating from his body, he was able to move forward with what happened next in the sequence of events. At this point, we used the Guardian Angel technique, asking for his grandmother to come in and provide love and nurturing for him and his twin. We also used the Guardian Angel technique for his adult self to tell him that it would all work out well, that he was loved, and that he was an incredible person.

All this was accomplished without my telling him that it was going to be okay and that he was safe. His guardian-angel grandmother happened to tell him that he was safe and so did his adult self. This is very acceptable and appropriate. What you need to realize is that *safe* is a No-No Word for *you* to use as a therapist.

Working with "safe"

If your client appears to be in distress or discomfort and you feel you need to do something, simply acknowledge it, verbally or nonverbally. Acknowledge it verbally by saying something like "It appears/seems to me that you are uncomfortable." (Own the observation. You will learn more about this in the next chapter, where we explore Wiggle Words.) Or you can ask an open-ended question such as "What do you need?" as opposed to a yes/no, closed-ended question like "Is there something you need?" (See chapter 7, "Open-Ended Questions versus Closed-Ended Questions" for a review of these types of questions.) Acknowledging what you notice is a simple and effective way to let your client know that she is being "presenced." Sometimes that is all that she needs—to be acknowledged.

Nonverbally you can acknowledge what is happening to your client by checking in with how grounded you are so that you are providing a solidly energetic safe space for her. If you are unsure about how to go about doing this, here are some basics to follow:[1]

- Make sure that you are breathing.

- Keep your feet on the floor.

- Maintain a clear understanding of what is your client's process and what is yours:
  - Be clear that you are not trying to "do" anything to your client.
  - Allow your client to have the experience; remember, you are an observer.
  - Do not energetically absorb or take on your client's difficulties.

You can also easily nonverbally acknowledge your client with a soft sound such as "Mmmm" or "Uh huhhh." Sometimes I even say something as simple as "Yup." These sounds send your client assurances that you are aware that something is going on. You may not know exactly what it is, but that is okay.

Once you have acknowledged your awareness of your client's distress or discomfort, simply wait for a response. She might reply immediately saying she is cold and needs a blanket. She might tell you that she remembered something very scary. She may not respond right away. A little time may pass before she says anything, if at all. In the time that passes, she might have worked through the situation on her own and not need anything else. Sometimes releases spontaneously occur just through the simple process of your client's becoming aware of something and both of you acknowledging and witnessing it. Then her body can let it go and move on to other things.

To recap: if your client appears to be in distress or discomfort:

- acknowledge—verbally or nonverbally

- say, "It appears/seems to me that you are uncomfortable." (Own the observation.)

- ask, "What do you need?" (OEQ versus "Is there something you need?" [Y/N])

- wait for a response from your client

Someone starts crying. What do you do? I had an interesting experience in one of my advanced CranioSacral Therapy and SomatoEmotional Release training classes. I was the client and was working on issues involving my mother and my soon-to-be ex-husband. I was at first just a little weepy and then tearful. One of

---

1   For more information about boundaries, grounding, and maintaining a therapeutic presence check out Suzanne Scurlock-Durana's "Healing from the Core" classes or other similar classes sponsored by various therapy schools and organizations.

my therapists, in this multiple-hand session, promptly got me a box of tissues and put some in my hand and started dabbing my wet cheeks and stroked my hair to soothe me. I felt so stifled and smothered. Inherently I knew that she did not mean to come across that way, but it was uncomfortable for me.

What do you do? Hand your crying client a tissue? The message conveyed is "There there, it'll be all right" or "It's okay; don't cry now." This is similar to saying, "You're safe; you're okay." What if she does not believe it will be all right, get better, or be okay? What if she was told as a child not to cry, to bite her lip, to buck up, that a big girl doesn't cry, not to show her emotions? Handing a tissue can be suppressive, stifling, and oppressive. It does not give her permission to experience her feelings. It does not give her permission to be with her awarenesses. Patting her hand, stroking her hair, and providing other "soothing" actions can communicate suppression. You want to avoid doing this.

Now for the rest of the story. After my session in the advanced class, during feedback time, I told my tissue-giving therapist how uncomfortable I felt when she dabbed away my tears and stroked my hair. As we discussed the situation, it was revealed that she was from Argentina. She did not know that, in American culture, this was not appropriate. In Argentina, what she had done was an expression of caring and was quite welcomed when done by a therapist. It was a great learning experience for all in the class. And I became even more aware of the importance of empowering my client to let me know what she needs.

What if your client really looks or acts as if she needs a tissue? It is as simple as acknowledging her by saying, "Let me know if you want a tissue at any time." As opposed to "Do you want a tissue?" which is a yes/no question. The question "Do you want a tissue?" is asking her what she wants at the current time, whereas if you say "At any time, just let me know…" she is given the power to choose when to ask for a tissue. Also asking her "Do you want a tissue?" can imply that she should stop crying because it is wrong to cry. This is clearly not the message that you want to convey.

OTHER CHOICE PHRASES

"How are you?"

I begin my SomaCentric Dialoguing classes by saying hello, welcoming and thanking the students for coming, and telling them how excited I am that they are there. I then tell them that I am going to ask them a question to which I want a one-word answer. I ask them, "How are you?" I write these answers on the easel pad and put tick marks next to the repeats. There are often a lot of repeated responses—"fine," "good," "tired." And some are more creative, like "excited," "on a horse" (energetic), "joyful," "tingly," "out of balance," and "hopeful."

Most responses are often trite and lack depth of meaning. A similar question—"How do you feel?"—quite often gets similar answers. "Good" and "fine" are very broad and general. These are quick responses or social scripts that we have learned to use. These really do not identify a client's state. "Good" or "fine" for one person may have an entirely different meaning to another. The response of "well" does not tell you if your client is feeling better than the last time she saw you or worse than how great she felt three days ago. Either asking a different question to start with or having your client elaborate on her response is necessary. If you ask a question other than "How are you?" you will get information quicker, and your sessions will progress easier.

You are looking for information. You are looking for broad information when your client comes in for his session, when he is experiencing something, and when his session is complete. If you want specific information, you need to avoid asking questions that will often be answered with a script such as "I'm fine."

When my client comes in, I may ask one of a couple of questions. If I ask "So what is going on?" he can tell me that he just got a raise, that he just had a fight, that he felt great for ten days after his last session, or that his foot now wants attention. "So what are we working on?" narrows the subject more specifically to what he wants help with and why he is there for a session. "What can I help you with?" gets a similar response.

After I acknowledge what my client has told me is going on, I ask the same question at the start of all sessions: "If there is one thing I can help you with today, what might that be?" I tell my client the first time I see him that I will always ask him this question. This empowers him to tell me that he wants help with a pulled shoulder from garden work or a bruised heel from standing on a cement floor too long or that his mother's dementia is getting worse and he wants some clarity over the reversal of the mother/son, nurturer/nurtured roles. This allows him to set his intention for the session, regardless of anything we have previously discussed in a treatment plan. If someone is coming to you for headaches but he sprained his wrist, his wrist very well may be a higher priority. Your client probably has coping mechanisms for the headaches, but he may not be able to function at work with a painful wrist, so that becomes his intention for the session.

I tell my client that I will ask at each session, "If there is one thing I can help you with today, what might that be?" also because knowing she will be asked this encourages her to start paying attention to her body prior to her session or the day before her session. The more she works with me, the more she pays attention and tries to answer this question. Some clients tell me that they start answering my question a few days before their session when they happen to be checking their schedule. I want this to happen. I want her listening to her body, and she does, whether she realizes it or not.

You want your client to give you information about what is happening with her body. You hope you have a good sense of what is going on, but it is her body and she is the expert. Instead of asking "How are you?" or "How do you feel?" have your client respond to a statement such as "Tell me what you are aware of." Since this is not a common directive, she does not have a ready-made response. When you have your client tell you what she notices, she has to pause and pay attention to what is going on in her body. This is the goal of SomaCentric Dialoguing: having the client pay attention and become more aware of what is happening in her body.

You want to educate your client and, in a sense, train her to become more aware of what is going on with her body. When your client responds with "I feel good," you can help her tune in with her body by asking her to describe that good feeling further. Ask, "What does 'good' feel like?" or "What is 'fine' like?" Or say, "Describe 'okay' to me."

At the end of a session, you want more information from your client. You want to know if you have helped her achieve the goal or intention she set at the beginning of the session. When she is fully present, if you ask "How do you feel?" she may give you a standard, pat answer. If so, ask, "What do you notice?" She has to notice how she is feeling. This question is not appropriately answered with "good." You hear, "My shoulders feel looser" or "My hand doesn't hurt as much." You can also ask, "What are you aware of?"

Taking it one step further, I have my client tell me about the changes that can happen in her life now that she is feeling a particular way. "Now that your body feels looser and more limber [how she previously defined what "good" feels like or what she noticed], what can happen differently in your life?" This helps her become more aware of the benefits of what can happen in her life when she pays attention and takes care of herself and her body.

If you pay attention to your word choice and change your questions, you will get lots of information. With this information, you can help your client be more in tune with her body, have information to help guide you as to what to do or ask next in the session, and educate your client that, when she takes care of herself, she can enjoy life more.

"Anything I should know about?"

Several skilled therapists have asked me the question above at the start of a session. The contrarian in me wanted defiantly to say, "Nope." The Brown part of me, short and to the point, wanted to say, "No." And yet I knew that they were looking for particular information.

This is one of the worst closed-ended questions that I have come across. It is easy for a client to say "No," when there in actuality is probably a lot about which you, the therapist, should know. Because it is a closed-ended question, it is not actually asking what you really want to know: "What should I know about, which you may or may not think is important to tell me, before I begin working with you?"

"Anything I should know about?" is a very broad question. The therapists who have asked this of me really wanted to ask, "What should I be aware of before I work with you, so that I can help you achieve your goals for this session?" Sometimes bodywork therapists ask this question hoping to clarify if there are any contraindications for the session. I, as a bodyworker, might know if a client's situation has a contraindication for a particular style of bodywork. However, this is not always the case. There are some styles of bodywork that have different contraindications. For example, a broken bone is not a contraindication for receiving CranioSacral Therapy or acupuncture. It is a contraindication for receiving Zero Balancing. A year after I started receiving Zero Balancing sessions, I learned and fully realized that broken bones were contraindications.

If my therapist had asked me "Anything I should know about?" and I had received an acupuncture session the week prior for a broken bone, I would not have known to say, "Oh, yeah, I broke…" If there is specific information for which you are searching, ask for it on your client intake form or ask your client directly before the session. "Have you broken any bones in the last three months?" will better give you the information you are seeking than "Anything I should know about?"

With regard to counseling sessions, "Anything I should know about?" is a seemingly pleasant way to inquire about what of significance has happened since the previous session. Again, it is easy for a client to say, "Nope." If you asked your client "What of significance has happened since your last session?" you would get much more specific information and be able to get more directly to the point.

If you are a Blue Success Signals communicator, it may feel uncomfortable being so direct by asking pointed questions and seeking specific information. When you are not in session, practice asking questions to yourself, a friend, or a colleague as if you were a Brown. Make a mental note about the client and situation when you catch yourself asking a question similar to "Anything I should know?" Rephrase your question, especially if you did not get the information you sought. If you do not have an appropriate opportunity to ask your question again, revisit it another time so that you are prepared for the next time. Through practicing rephrasing, you will discover a couple of different ways to ask your question.

FRIENDLY REMARKS

The next concept that I am going to present is something for you to consider in general. Pay attention to how it plays out in your sessions and your general communication with your clients. It is an example of how what you say, depending upon the words you choose, can mean different things.

Years ago, my mother told me about getting her colors analyzed. She was not referring to the Success Signals communication styles described in this book. She was referring to seasonal-color analysis as is described in Carole Jackson's book *Color Me Beautiful*. She had her colors analyzed so that she could know what colors of clothes and makeup were more flattering for her to wear. For a birthday present, she gave me the gift of a consultation so that I could have my colors analyzed. I was not interested in the makeup because I did not wear it, but I was intrigued by why I liked certain clothing colors and not others.

Here is one of the most profound comments the consultant told me. After she determined that I was a Winter, she asked me if I had ever said to a friend, "I like the blouse you have on." I acknowledged that I had. She told me that this could be interpreted two ways. First, I could be saying, "I really like the color of your blouse; that would look good on me." Second, I could be saying, "The color of your blouse really looks good on you. You should wear that color more often." With the first interpretation, I was making a statement about myself and what would be flattering to me. With the second interpretation, I was making a statement that is about how flattering the color was on my friend.

How does this all relate to SomaCentric Dialoguing? It is an example of how a seemingly simple and benign statement like "I like the blouse you have on" can actually be interpreted to mean two different things: one about me and one about my friend. The same could be said about when you give comments and compliments about:

- the car a person drives: are you indicating that you would like to be driving that car, or are you saying that the car is appropriate for the other person?

- a piece of art or the way a room is decorated: are you indicating that you would like that in your home, or are you complimenting your friend on how well it fits with the rest of her décor?

- the way her hair is styled: are you indicating that you think the style would look good on you, or are you telling her how flattering it looks for her face?

When you have a client in the office, you have to make sure that the focus is on your client. If you like the sweater or the piece of jewelry she is wearing because you think it would look good on you, be careful what you say. If you think her sweater or her jewelry is flattering to her, acknowledge it: "That sweater looks flattering on you." One caveat is that you need to be careful about therapeutic relationships and boundaries. Avoid creating a situation where your client tries to dress for each session to please you. This can possibly lead to countertransference problems.

If I do compliment a client it is for a good reason, not just to make them feel good. It is not my job to make my client feel good. I generally will not compliment a client unless I have been working with them for an extended period of time. If my client's physical appearance seems to be improving, as exhibited by a sparkle in her eye or an increase in vitality, I might cautiously acknowledge what I see. (For more information about transference and countertransference, I recommend that you read Nina McIntosh's *The Educated Heart*.)

HUMOR

Often humor and laughter can be quite helpful to relax your client and help release tension. He can use it to get in touch with what is going on in his body and to realize how a perception is irrationally viewed or held. This being said, sometimes what one person thinks is funny, another does not find humorous. I generally do not make jokes with my client until he has introduced humor. I let him show me his humor language and let him make us both laugh.

Red communicators often love humor. When dialoguing, a Red is apt to express what is happening in his body with lots of flair. When he does this, it is okay to laugh with him. If you are not comfortable laughing, instead of a laugh, use a big smile. By nature, I am a Brown communicator. Occasionally, I can tell a good joke, but it does not always come easily. So I let my client take the lead. It is all about him anyway. And, even then, I only joke with him a little and only for therapeutic purposes.

When in an altered state, the subconscious has no place for humor. In addition to using caution with humor, please avoid irony and sarcasm. These are sometimes difficult to perceive correctly and are especially challenging to perceive when a client is in an altered state. Teasing is not humorous and is never appropriate. It is often confused with irony and sarcasm. Many emotional scars have been left by the blade of teasers, and you do not want to add to your client's collection. Completely avoid any teasing, even if your client starts it.

AVOID SEX, RELIGION, POLITICS, AND MONEY

When SomaCentric Dialoguing with clients, use extreme clarity and heightened awareness when your client brings up topics of sex, religion, politics, and money. There are too many boundaries that could be potentially crossed or expressions that could be misconstrued. If you do not know your client's religious or political preferences you could easily offend your client. This could lead also to a poor reputation within your community. Any discussion about sex could be misconstrued to imply a sexual attraction, of which your client might take offense or inappropriately make unwanted sexual advances toward you. An awkward power differential could be created when discussing money. Depending upon the conversation about money, your client may feel that you are financially well off and therefore believe that you are charging them too much.

All of these situations create unnecessary awkwardnesses that can be avoided easily by not bringing up the subject. If a client does bring up one of these subjects it is acceptable to say something as simple and straightforward as "I do not discuss [awkward subject] with my clients." Follow up this statement with a question or statement that focuses the session back to the client and his therapeutic needs. Play it safe and avoid these conversations. Once again, I refer you to McIntosh's *The Educated Heart*, where more information about the hazards of these discussions is presented.

DEADLY WORD CHOICES

Sometimes the words you use in everyday language can have an unrealized negative effect on your health. I call these words "deadly." One day, I was talking with a good friend about his ex-wife and conversations that they have repeatedly. He said to me, "Julie, it just kills me every time she says something like that." I asked him to stop and think about the message that he sent his body every time he said, "It kills me." I pointed out to him that he was giving his body permission to harm himself when his ex-wife would say hurtful things.

The phrase "It pains me" carries similar connotations. Words carry energy and intention. Many studies and books have been written confirming this. In particular, medical intuitive and motivational speaker Carolyn Myss talks about this in many of her books and presentations (see bibliography).

I spent the afternoon with a dear friend who kept telling me, "I'm falling apart." What she was really trying to tell me is that her life was not as easeful as she would like it. I reflected back to her what she was saying. We discussed how what she was telling her body and her life was that she did not have things together, when in actuality she had a pretty good life, but she wanted the different aspects of her life to be working more smoothly. By continually telling herself, me, and others, "I'm falling apart," she reinforced the concept that she did not have things together.

Another phrase of Deadly Words that I often hear and even used to say myself is "I can't believe it!" It is a common phrase often used when something good happens to you. When you say "I can't believe it!" you are telling your body that it is too good to be true and, therefore, you should not acknowledge that this is actually occurring. Do you want to believe it? Or not? If you do, then celebrate what is happening—"I'm so excited and happy!" is a much truer and more accurate reflection of what is meant.

When I hear a client using a word or phrase that she really does not mean, especially something that could be considered a Deadly Word, I help her understand the message that she is actually communicating. I invite you to do the same.

As you go through your daily personal and professional life, pay attention to the word choices that you are making. What messages are you sending your clients? What are you really asking them? What messages are you telling your body and yourself? Pay attention to your word choice. By avoiding the use of No-No Words, dialoguing with your clients will improve. Avoid using Deadly Words, and your body and your life will be healthier.

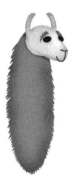

By the way, did you know that *Roget's Thesaurus* has 38 synonyms for the word pain?

Oh my! I wonder what my client really means.

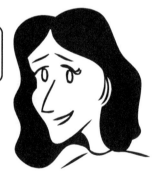

9 Wiggle Words

Own your statements! Do it with Wiggle Words! In the previous chapter on word choice, I mentioned that what your client says is important. What *you*, the therapist, say is possibly more important. Throughout the session, from the time your client arrives to the time she leaves, there will be opportunities when you need to restate or reframe something she has said. It is imperative for you to own your words. Own your words with Wiggle Words!

"Wiggle Words"—what do I mean by this? The purpose of Wiggle Words is to have a way to reframe a client's statement, ask a question, or share an impression, and at the same time put the onus of being wrong on yourself, while giving the client permission to change, add, alter, or deny what you have said.

Imagine this scenario. Your client looks uncomfortable, and the room feels a little chilly to you. If you say to a client "You look cold. Would you like a blanket?" she may have a difficult time correcting you if she is not cold. Something else may be going on that makes her look uncomfortable. She may not feel comfortable enough to tell you that you are wrong. If you use Wiggle Words, you can make it easier for your client to feel comfortable telling you that you are wrong. "It seems to me that you are cold. Would you like a blanket?" is a gentler way to tell her what you are observing.

She might actually be okay and just try to figure something out. Do not assume you know what is going on inside the client. Using Wiggle Words is an easy way to give her permission to say, "No, I just have an itch that needs scratching."

Wiggle Words allow your words to be received softly and gently when you restate or reframe something your client has said. The power behind Wiggle Words comes when you take responsibility and ownership of any observation, and it provides your client with the opportunity to tell you that you are off-track or inaccurate or wrong.

It is vital to own the statement. Make sure to use an "I" statement. If you say "It seems as if..." then you are supposing you know what your client means and are not owning the statement yourself. If you say "It seems to me," then you are owning the statement. It may initially sound like just a minor difference of semantics, but when you start to work with Wiggle Words, you will notice a difference.

The next time you have a casual conversation with someone, maybe at lunch or dinner, try some Wiggle Words with your statements. Tell him what you are learning and get his feedback as to how it feels with the different statements. Then, try it with your clients, and notice the difference in their energy and response.

Wiggle Words are important for all therapists to use. If you happen to be like me, a strong Brown communicator who is inclined to just say it how it is, Wiggle Words can help you soften how you dialogue with clients. Your Blue clients will especially like this.

Here is a list of good Wiggle Words and phrases. This list is not all inclusive, and I encourage you to think of your own:

- possibly

- perhaps

- Would I be correct to say...?

- It seems to me... (versus "It looks/seems like"—not owned)

- It appears to me... (versus "It appears as if"—appears to whom? Not owned)

- Correct me if I'm wrong...

- Correct me if I'm inaccurate...

- If this resonates with you...

- maybe, maybe not

- How about...?

- What if...?

- Would it be fair to say...

- This is what I'm hearing/seeing/sensing...

- Help me out here.

- Change what doesn't work for you.

Often I string a number of these Wiggle Words and phrases together to impress upon my client how inaccurate I might be and to invite him to correct me or change anything. For you to get a better understanding of this concept and how it works, here are some Wiggle Word statements with the different components analyzed:

It seems to me, and feel free to correct me if I'm inaccurate, that [insert your observation].

- "It seems" are disclaimer Wiggle Words

- "to me" shows ownership, that it is your observation, not the client's

- "feel free to correct me" gives your client permission to correct what you say

- "if I'm" again shows your ownership of the observation

- "inaccurate" again tells your client he is allowed to tell you that you are wrong

Please let me know if this resonates with you, what I hear is [insert your observation].

- "Please let me know" empowers your client to tell you something one way or the other

- "if this resonates with you" asks your client if your observation is correct

- "what I hear is" indicates your ownership of your observation

Correct me if I'm wrong, but it seems to me, and tell me if I'm off base, that [insert your observation].

- "Correct me if I'm wrong" empowers your client to tell you that you are wrong

- "it seems to me" shows you are taking ownership of your observation

- "tell me if I'm off base" again acknowledges to your client that it is acceptable for her to say, "Nope, you got it wrong"

It seems to me, and change my words if I've gotten it wrong, I am sensing that [insert your statement].

- "It seems" are disclaimer Wiggle Words

- "to me" is your ownership of what you are about to reflect back to your client

- "and change my words" gives your client permission to make your statement accurate

- "I am sensing" is your ownership of your statement

> It seems to me—and please correct me if I'm wrong—that perhaps you are getting a good sense of how Wiggle Words are important in SomaCentric Dialoguing.

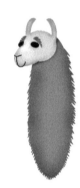

The formula for using Wiggle Words is the following:

1. Start with a disclaimer Wiggle Word(s) such as "it seems," "possibly," or "perhaps."

2. Add in some words of ownership of your statement or observation, such as "to me" and "I."

3. Put in some words of permission for your client to tell you that you are inaccurate and to give him permission to change what you have said.

4. Finish with your observation, statement, restatement, or reframing of what your client has said or done.

WIGGLE WORDS EXERCISE

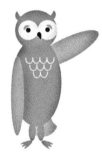

How many more Wiggle Words or phrases can you think of?

How many Wiggle Word sentences can you think of?

10 *Getting Started*

You are now at the point where you have learned the fundamentals of dialoguing. You have learned about the importance of holding a safe space, what it means to be a facilitator, what the cause of various problems can be, how to determine what is a yes-or-no question, and how important it is to have your client speak in first person and present tense. Additionally, you have learned about two different language styles: the Success Signals color communication styles and audial, visual, and kinesthetic (AVK) processing styles. You have learned about why a client may not want or does not know how to dialogue and how to work with those impediments productively. Now it is time to put these all together and to get started with your dialoguing sessions.

You need to start somewhere and quite often the easiest place to start is where your hands are on your client. The technique "How to Get Started," as described here, is designed for therapists who do hands-on therapy. Those who do not do hands-on sessions should simply modify the first part, as described further in this chapter. Sometimes the process of getting started is the most awkward. Once you start rolling with the dialoguing, it gets easier. This technique is just one way to begin. Use it as a guide and feel free to alter it to suit your therapeutic style. You will find additional helpful information about how to create and start sessions in chapter 13, "Creating a Session."

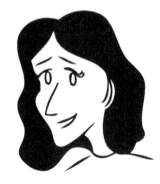

Are you ready to try what you have learned so far?

HOW TO GET STARTED TECHNIQUE

1. Place your hands on your client in the area he has identified.

    This area may be one that causes him some discomfort or distress. If he is unable to identify an area to start with, use any tools and techniques that you have to listen to the body to determine where to start working first. It does not always mean that, when you start in one particular place, this place is the source of your client's problem.

2. With your hands on your client, ask him to bring his awareness to your hands.

    This helps him to focus on one spot. Quite often the vastness of his body can distract him from paying attention to one specific area. It is your job, as the therapist, to help him focus his awareness in one starting location.

3. Pause and allow him a few moments to focus his awareness.

4. Ask him to get a good *sense* of that area.

    Use the word sense *because you want him to use all his processing styles when he tunes in with what is going on in his body. As you continue to have him become aware and later on describe what he is aware of, then you can use words that are part of his AVK processing language.*

5. Pause and allow him a few moments to get a sense of the area under your hands.

6. Ask him to get a good sense of what is or is not going on in that area.

    You want to encourage him to stay here in this one place. Sometimes nothing is actually happening; there is a lack of something. This is significant. *Anything that catches his attention is important at this point.*

7. Pause to allow him to sense what is going on.

8. Ask him to *notice* where his attention is being drawn.

   Again, this is to keep him focused in his body. You want to use the word notice *to cover all the AVK processing styles. It may seem redundant to repeat over and over again that you want him to pay attention to the area under your hands. Repeat your request many times. Repeat it in slightly different ways to help deepen his awareness.*

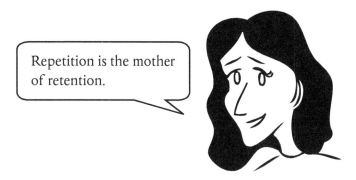

Repetition is the mother of retention.

(From here on, the technique also works for a hands-off session. See the "Hands off?" section below for more information.)

9. Again, pause to give him time.

   These pauses do not need to be long. Sometimes I pause for 10 to 15 seconds, sometimes up to a minute. The length of the pause depends upon what I, as the therapist, am aware is going on with the client. I continue when my Indicator Compass indicates that my client is aware of something significant or that he is on track.

10. Say, "Let me know when you have a good sense of it."

    Have him give you an indication that he can articulate something about the area of his body that you have asked him to sense and notice.

11. When you get acknowledgment that he has a good sense of the area, ask him, "What are you aware of?"

    This is an all-important, open-ended question. Be sure it is well worded. Avoid using the words think, know, figure out. *Words such as these bring your client into thinking mode, which is something that you want to avoid. His brain/mind has had a multitude of opportunities to tell him what the brain thinks about the body part. Now is your client's opportunity to get the message directly from the body part in question.*

When you ask this question, use the word aware *or* notice *instead of* think, know, *or* figure out, *which you may accidentally say from habit.*

12.   From here, just follow his trail of what he tells you.

The purpose of this technique is to help your client become aware of what his body wants to tell him. From here, use the key concepts, proper word choice, and lots of Wiggle Words to help him get the message that his body wants to communicate. Use his AVK processing style, if you know it, to help him clarify this message. Also use the various other techniques to help your client achieve the goal set at the beginning of the session.

When your client gets stuck, offer him suggestions with lots of Wiggle Words, as described in the preceding chapter. For example:

"Get a good sense of what it looks like, what it sounds like, what it feels like."

"If it were to have a <u>color</u>, what would it be?"

"If it were to have a <u>shape</u>, what would it be?"

Fill in the blanks with a variety of adjectives, such as:

- texture to touch
- size
- smell
- temperature
- sound
- name

What other adjectives can you think of?

Hands off?

Are you a therapist who is not a bodyworker? Perhaps you are a psychotherapist or counselor of some sort, an athletic trainer, or even someone who works via phone consultations. You do not put your hands on your client, nor do you have her lay on a massage table. This same SomaCentric Dialoguing work can be done with your hands off a seated client. If you have a couch for her to lay on, that also works. The hands-off therapy begins in a slightly different way from the hands-on technique, but, after the first two steps, it employs the same methods.

1.   For non-hands-on sessions, start with your client's taking some deep, full breaths.

This helps bring her focus and attention into her body. You could also ask her to close her eyes while she does this to help her better center her attention and avoid visual distractions. This is particularly helpful for those who are visual processors. You can ask your client to put her hands on the area of her body that she initially is aware of to help focus her attention on her body.

2. Ask her to pay attention to her body as she breathes deeply.

Have your client notice where her attention is drawn as she breathes. The obvious answer might seem that she would automatically focus on her lungs or ribs because she is breathing deeply. This is not always the case. Quite often, her attention will be drawn to an area of her body that bothers her or wants some attention. Have her put her hands on that area of her body. This may be the same area or a different one than initially. It is okay for her to move her hands. If the body part cannot be reached, she can image her hands there.

From here, it is just as if your client were lying on a table. Follow the rest of the directions of the preceding section, steps 9 through 12.

How to Get Started, Abbreviated Version

To review, here is "How to Get Started" again, but in an abbreviated version. This is the hands-on version. Feel free to adjust the instructions, as described previously, if you do not do hands-on work.

1. With your hands on the client, ask him to bring his awareness to where your hands are.

2. Ask him to get a good sense of that area.

3. Ask him to get a good sense of what is or is not going on in that area.

4. Ask him to notice where his attention is being drawn.

5. Ask him to let you know when he has a good sense.

6. When you get acknowledgment that he has a good sense of the area, ask him, "What are you aware of?"

7. Now just follow the trail he gives you.

8. If he gets stuck, offer him suggestions with lots of Wiggle Words:

   • "Get a good sense of what it looks like, what it sounds like, what it feels like."

   • "If it were to have a <u>color</u>, what would it be?"

   • "If it were to have a <u>shape</u>, what would it be?"

   • texture to touch

- size

- smell

- temperature

- sound

- name

PERMISSION TECHNIQUE

There are many reasons and opportunities to use the Permission technique, one of my favorites. I like it so much because it is simple and easy to use. I invite you to play with it, with your clients and even with yourself. Be creative with when and where you use it.

The Permission technique is great to use when it seems that your client is stuck and not getting anywhere. As discussed earlier, many clients have never been given permission to be aware of what was going on in their body, which can lead to a multitude of problems. Recently, a client, Sally, was referred to me by a colleague. Sally had told my colleague that, after 60 years, she was tired of keeping things held inside and not dealing with them: "It's about time I did something about it!" We used the Permission technique to help Sally do something about her repression.

Use the Permission technique when a client has previously pushed aside a feeling or an aspect of herself or she has not allowed herself to experience a particular emotion. Quite often underlying health problems—whether physical, nutritional, or emotional—can be caused by a client's never having been given permission to acknowledge, be aware of, and feel that part of herself. This was the case with Patricia, as I described earlier in chapter 6, the chapter on dialoguing.

If you reach a certain point while trying to meet a client's particular objective, such as determining why her hip is painful, and she cannot get in touch with that area, the Permission technique can help her. Or if you have repeatedly used other techniques resulting in little headway or diminishing progress, try the Permission technique. It can help the client break through plateaus in her healing.

Permission is very helpful when a client continually goes off track, drifts out of her body, or talks in circles. You can help her come back into her body-centered awareness by using the Permission technique because it provides your client with a structured opportunity to come back into her body and get back on track. Below are the steps for the Permission technique:

1. Hold a safe space.

    If necessary, please refresh yourself with what was previously discussed in chapter 2 about holding a safe space. If your client experiences a sensitive situation for the first time or the first time in a long time, she may be uncomfortable or unsure. A safe and supportive environment is very important for her. At some point, your client may grimace, or some tears may roll down her cheeks. This is okay. Allow it to happen. Continue to hold a safe space for her.

2. Give your client permission to feel what she is aware of.

    Here you provide her with something that she may never have had: permission to experience, feel, or be aware of an emotion, feeling, or part of herself.

3. Say, "Get a good sense of that area of your body."

    Encourage her to get a good sense of "it," the part of her body that has gotten her attention. Whatever "it" actually is may not always be important. Her sense and awareness of it is what is important.

4. Pause…pause…pause.

    Pause between statements. Allow the client the opportunity to do what you have asked—get a sense of her body. This is when you need to start paying attention to what happens to your client and within her body without relying on her words. Go back to the section "Indicator Compass—Determining 'yes' or 'no'" in chapter 3, "Key Concepts." Tune your radar into what is going on in her body, using your tracking system. It is okay if this takes some practice. Know that you will not hurt your client if you are not able to track every nuance of her experiences. Keep with this format and you will do fine.

5. Say, "Just give yourself permission to be with it."

    Now it is time to give her, perhaps for the first time, permission to tune in with herself.

6. Say, "Just be with it."

    You are giving her permission to be with it. Her being with it is more important than anything else at this point of the session.

7. Pause for a while. Pay attention to what is going on with her.

8. Say, "Give yourself permission."

    It may seem funny to tell someone something that seems so obvious. However, when your client is in a semialtered state, the obvious does need to be stated. So, state it.

9. Say, "Give yourself permission to be with *that*."

    It may seem unnecessary to be redundant. Like stating the obvious, when your client is in a semialtered state, she can start drifting off to la-la land. Or she can go off on a different tangent, and you might not know it because she does not tell you what is going on. Repeat instructions clearly and simply to keep her on track.

10.   Say, "Get a good sense of it."

Yes, you are repeating yourself now. Get used to it. When you change a few words, but keep the message the same, you help her to go deeper into her awareness.

11.   Say, "Yup. Just be there."

12.   Say, "Stay with it."

Repeat these or similar lines. These lines can be spoken in any order. I start with a statement that specifically has the word permission *in it. Keep what you say to a minimum, and insert many long pauses between your gently directive phrases.*

At first, you may be overly wordy, and that is okay. Just try a briefer sentence next time.

When she gets a good sense of "it" and she has given herself permission to be fully with it, feel it, see it, touch it, etc., then you can move on to have her explore the message that part of her wants to communicate.

When are you done?

The Permission technique is complete when your client has achieved the awareness or information that he needed for that part of his session. Your client's realization may be the solution to an issue. It may be the piece that was necessary for him to move on to some other part of the session. It may seem that he needed to experience permission in order to feel something before a block or resistance could be resolved.

Follow the lead of your client. Have no agenda regarding what the outcome should be. You may be sitting there very quietly, helping your client just be with part of himself, and the next thing that happens is he is vivaciously describing a huge awareness. This technique is about helping your client connect to himself and gain an awareness or realization. Once he has his realization, continue in the direction your client takes. The session may end quietly with a big sigh, which indicates he has reached the realization that he needed.

How to make permission effective

The key to this technique's being so highly effective is that you do *not* have your client describe her awareness. By not describing what she now feels, she is free just to experience what is going on in her body. To put words to an experience can sometimes be a struggle and a distraction. The Permission technique is about experiencing and being aware of what is happening in her body. When words are used to describe the situation, the client shifts from body-awareness to a thinking mode. This needs to be avoided. Assist your client to remain in body-centered awareness.

If your client feels moved to say something, that is okay. However, a slight note of caution: if it seems that she tries to keep you informed of her awarenesses, then encourage her to wait until later to speak. This is easily done by saying, "Thank you, but I do not need you to tell me right now what is going on. I'd like you just to be with your body [or name the specific area if you are aware of it] right now. If I need you to put words to anything, I will let you know." If she tells you what she is aware of because she needs help, then assist her. Pay attention to any talk that may indicate that she is avoiding being aware of what is happening in her body (resistance). Evaluate the situation and refocus her attention on giving herself permission to be with her body sensations and messages.

When you use the Permission technique, refrain from asking questions. If it is necessary to ask a question, make it very specific and brief. It is easier to ask very succinct questions about the client's experience if you speak her language (communication and/or processing style). After you have asked a question, make sure you help her return to her body-centered awareness.

Keep your statements brief and vague. Do not delve into the realm of having the client sense a color, size, texture, shape, or other attribute of that area of her body. This technique is all about allowing her just to be with a particular part of her body. A teacher of mine once said that it is like sitting in the mud with your client. There is nothing to do, nothing to say, nothing to feel. It is just mud in which she is stuck. When you think about it, it is amazing what can come out of the mud.

I hope you had the opportunity as a kid to sit in the mud. Let me extend this wonderful metaphor. Remember back to a time when you were out playing in the rain and you slipped. Plop! Down you went. Much to your mother's chagrin, not only were you wet, but you were now also muddy. Maybe the fall hurt or caught you by surprise. Now you are all muddy, and there is nothing you can do about it. Or is there?

There is something you can do about it! You can sit there in the mud and just be muddy and wet. As you notice the mud on your hands, legs, and shirt, you have an awareness. You understand a fundamental concept. You realize, as you sit in the mud, that mud is great to throw and get others muddy! Now your problem and your pain have instantaneously been turned into a great "Aha!" moment, accompanied by a mischievous grin as you prepare to get your sister just as muddy as you.

I invite you to sit in the mud, proverbial or real, with your client. You are there to give her permission to be there. Give her permission to be there in her body. There is nothing to figure out. Eventually, as she becomes more in touch with her body, she will have more awarenesses. Perhaps she will sit there wallowing in the mire. Keep her sitting there. Give her permission to remain there. Encourage her just to sit in that mud. She does not have to figure out anything, just be there. Make sure she does not start to talk and analyze the situation. At some point, you will notice her energy shift and her breathing may change. Tears may come or a smile may crack as she realizes something. That something is the essence of SomaCentric Dialoguing.

Identifying "it"

I want to discuss identifying "it." "It" refers to a body sensation or part that your client has been given permission to notice. What I mean by "identifying" is the actual naming of that place in his body upon which he is focused. I have found that sometimes it is very helpful to identify "it," using a statement like "Just be with the area under your rib."

Identifying "it" is advantageous because this helps focus your client on a very specific part or region of his body. When you identify "it," use the word or term that your client used. Hearing his own words spoken empowers him to be in touch with himself and reinforces the Permission technique. If you do not identify "it," your client may have a little more difficulty focusing on a particular part of his body. By not identifying "it," he may be more prone to floating off and not being in his body.

And yet there is a catch; sometimes identifying "it" can slow the progress of the session. If the situation or problem that your client actually needs to focus his awareness on is not the area identified, he may get distracted and not pay attention. This can happen even if the client has consciously identified "it" previously, as is discussed below. So, an advantage of not identifying "it" is that sometimes the area the client thinks he is supposed to be focusing on is not the actual area he needs to pay attention to; in this situation, his subconscious has an easier time bringing his awareness to the actual part upon which he needs to focus if the conscious mind is not hearing the first body part restated by the therapist.

How do you balance the two? I suggest that you initially identify "it" one or maybe two times. When you progress further with the Permission technique, stop using the identifier. Initially, you will be helping him to focus his attention on that area of the body. When you stop naming that particular part of his body, his conscious and subconscious awarenesses can communicate without being distracted by being drawn continually to the identified area.

This concept of identifying "it," like many aspects of SomaCentric Dialoguing, is not taught to therapists. Usually, it takes years of astute practice to notice when or not and how or not to do something. Learn this fact now, and you can leap ahead of the usual learning curve!

Yes, but…

Somewhere along the way, your client may tell you "That's not really the part of my body that wants my attention. It is my _____." If this happens, thank her for telling you. Encourage her to explore the area that needs her attention. Please do not disagree with her. She knows her body better than anyone else. She is in the middle of processing something significant and important.

I have observed practice sessions where the client told the therapist a little background, stated what she wanted to work on, and named a part of the body as the possible source of the problem. Let us use the shoulder for this example. It happened like this:

> *Therapist to client*: Give yourself permission to get in touch with your shoulder.
>
> *Pause*
>
> *Therapist*: Get a good sense of it.
>
> *Pause*
>
> *Therapist*: Just be with your shoulder.
>
> *Pause*
>
> *Client*: Actually, it's not my shoulder; it is my back.
>
> *Therapist*: Give yourself permission to be aware of your shoulder.
>
> *Client*: It really seems like my back is trying to get my attention.
>
> *Therapist*: Thank your back, and let it know that you'll pay attention to it later. Now bring your focus back to your shoulder because that was where you initially located the problem.
>
> *The client complies after an awkward pause because the therapist is supposed to know what to do.*

At this point, I politely asked if I could pause the session and offer some fine-tuning. Both the client and the therapist agreed. I reflected back the client's words to the therapist. I explained that it was the client's inner knowing or inner wisdom that was trying to show the client that the shoulder was not the problem, even though there seemingly might be some very good reason for that part of the body to be the cause of the problem. However, the client's back was the place that the body actually wanted the awareness and attention.

As a therapist, you need to remove yourself from the picture. Set aside your own agenda or ideas about how your client's healing should happen and what it should look like. The most knowledgeable therapist for your client is her own body. Your job is only to facilitate that communication between your client and her body. Sometimes you may get superseded by your client's body butting in and shouting, "Hey! Hey, you! Hey, blockhead—it's your back that is causing the pain! Not your shoulder."

This is exactly what you want to happen, believe it or not! SomaCentric Dialoguing is all about helping your client get in touch with what is happening in her body so she can heal herself. When this happens, you have successfully done your job. Here is a "high five" to both your client and you.

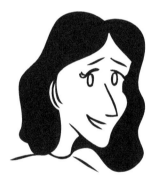

Key concepts for the Permission technique:
- Don't interrupt your client with questions of descriptions of her awareness.
- Don't ask her details.
- Just be supportive and encouraging.

MINI ME TECHNIQUE

The Mini Me technique is a great way to start a dialoguing session. If the concept of becoming aware of his body is new to your client, this helpful technique introduces him to the concept of tuning in to his body. Use this technique when a client has a difficult time finding the area of his body that is trying to get his attention. Use his communication and processing languages to maximize the effectiveness of this technique.

This is a great way to help a client start to become at ease with visualizing, sensing, or pretending something in a manner that he might not be comfortable with. Sometimes a client who is predominantly a Brown or a Green and more comfortable thinking and rationalizing about how things happen has more resistance to going with the process. When a client has a very difficult time and tells me that he believes he is "just making it up," I invite him to think of Mr. Rogers' Neighborhood of Make-Believe. Quite often this gets a smile or even a laugh from him and helps him relax. Mr. Rogers' Neighborhood of Make-Believe, or the land of make-believe, is a familiar concept to all. At some point in my client's life, playing pretend may have been meaningful. I ask my client to "just imagine" and give it a try. After he tries it, he is often pleased and amazed with the results.

The script I use with my clients

I want you to imagine reducing yourself to a mini-size.

Maybe you will use a machine similar to the one in the movie *Honey, I Shrunk the Kids*.

Or maybe you will use a special pill.

Or you simply may see or feel yourself getting smaller and smaller until you are a Mini Me.

Pause

Let me know when you are mini in size.

Pause

Once you are very small, I want you to find a way to get into your body.

Perhaps crawl in through your ear.

Melt and be absorbed into your skin.

Walk into your mouth and slide down…

Or you might just imagine yourself automatically shrinking into the center of your body.

Whatever works for you, use it to get inside yourself.

Pause

When you are inside yourself, let me know.

Pause

Now I want you to explore inside yourself.

Walk around.

Float around.

Feel where you are naturally drawn.

Pause

Find a place in your body that needs attention.

Allow your Mini Me to go to the place in your body that is wanting attention.

There may be a few places to which you are drawn.

If so, find the area that draws you most strongly.

Pause

If you need a flashlight to light your way, realize you have one in your hand already.

If you need a map to follow, it's in your pocket.

If you need a sign to show you, look up; it is right there.

Pause

Give your Mini Me permission to go wherever your body wants attention.

Pause

When you get to the area trying to get your attention, let me know.

Client indicates she is there.

Okay…

Now get a good sense of what is around you.

Pause

Where are you?

What are you aware of?

Tell me more…

Continue from this point of awareness having the client describe that area of her body. Use dialoguing to have her become aware of the message or reason that area of her body wants attention.

1-2-3 TECHNIQUE

Use the 1-2-3 technique when your client has difficulty trusting what she is aware of or has a difficult time finding a starting place. In chapter 12, "Gems and Nuances," I describe the importance of flash-pan thoughts. Briefly, a flash-pan thought is the first thing that comes to mind when asked a question. In "Gems and Nuances," I discuss why first impressions can be trusted and are valid. Use the first thing that comes to your client's awareness as this is often significant. It may not be the most important thing, but it can be an entry point into the body. Use your client's first awareness as a helpful way to begin dialoguing with the situation that needs to be addressed. The answer may or may not be a particular body part. The first awareness may be an emotion or a memory. Remember there are no right or wrong answers. The purpose of this technique is to help your client trust her body's responses and to establish a starting point for a dialoguing session.

Simple instructions to give your client

I want you to close your eyes and just start noticing your body in general.

Take some deep breaths in and out.

As you breathe, notice your entire body as a whole, inside and out.

I'm going to count to three.

On three, you are going to tell me the first thing that pops up in your mind,

the first thing that comes into your awareness.

I want you just to go with it.

Allow the first thought to enter your mind without analyzing, censoring, or filtering it.

So, on three...

One,

Brief pause; then in a little firmer tone

Two,

Brief pause; then in an even firmer tone with authority

Three!

Pay attention to your Indicator Compass so you can help your client track if she is censoring her first response, should she try consciously or subconsciously not to acknowledge her first response.

What did you notice?

Tell me more.

Through dialoguing, help your client explore what she noticed. Make sure to validate her experience by acknowledging that trusting the process might have been difficult. Using lots of Wiggle Words, help her connect the dots between her intention for the session and whatever her body wanted her to be aware of with this technique.

10 THINGS TECHNIQUE

Use the 10 Things technique when a client has a difficult time describing what he senses. Ask your client to describe ten things about the area that he wants to explore. This is a quick and easy way to start a SomaCentric Dialoguing session. It can be used when you are not sure how to help your client begin dialoguing. Additionally, use the 10 Things technique if your client has a difficult time determining the message his body wants to communicate. This technique can be done in a short period of time, in only 5 to 15 minutes.

Ideally, descriptions should consist of only one or two words to keep the client's awareness in that area of his body and to prevent him from shifting into his head. You want to avoid having him analyze or rationalize his awarenesses. Keep the descriptions brief to help keep your client focused on his body. If he gives you more than a couple of words while he describes his ten things, politely interrupt him and instruct him that you want him to use only one or two words for each description.

Inform your client that you will keep count of how many descriptors he gives you. As he gives you his list, pay attention to what he says and the order in which he gives his responses. (It is okay to take notes.) In addition to keeping count, after he has said some things, repeat some of them back to him. (See example below.) Usually by the fourth description, he will take a pause as he searches for the next description. When appropriate, repeat back in the same order what he has said and let him know how many descriptions he has provided.

As the client proceeds, repeat back to him one word of the description he has just said. As you keep track of the number of descriptions, tell him how many he has told you, as well as how many more he has to go. If he gets stuck, repeat back in the order given a number of his descriptions. Encourage the client and help him stay focused on his body if he seems to get distracted or into his head.

As he tells you ten descriptions of the area upon which he is focusing, the client gets deeper into his process and body-centered awareness.

When he gets to his tenth, repeat the tenth description and then pause. Next, instruct him to give you one more description, an eleventh. This is the most important description. It is the one that was lying beyond the qualities, experiences, and issues of which he was conscious. Quite often this is one he may have tried unconsciously to avoid telling you. This eleventh one is the one that you will have him explore in the session. The other ten descriptions are valid but are less significant than his eleventh description.

Once he has given you his eleventh description, use the dialoguing skills and techniques in this book to help your client explore the significance of this final description.

Generally, I have found that Reds and Blues will have an easier time describing what they are feeling. Emotions will be evident in their expressions more quickly than in those of Browns or Greens. Browns and Greens will be more apt to give facts, rather than describe emotions or feelings.

An example

Therapist: I want you to describe for me ten things about your shoulder.

The client may start with basic and obvious adjectives of her shoulder.

Client: It's boney.

It's hard to the touch.

It's white-colored.

It feels tight.

And then the client pauses. The first four are easy. Now she starts trying to figure out how else to describe her shoulder.

Your repeating back to her what she has said does a couple of things for your client. It acknowledges that you have heard her. By hearing her own words, it deepens her awareness of her shoulder. Repeating back while she is searching for the next descriptions helps her to brainstorm for the next word. It is important to repeat back what she has said in the same order. Use her words. It is acceptable to use only one word, shortening her descriptions.

Therapist: (*You repeat back to her*) It's boney.

It's hard.

White.

Tight.

That's four.

Keep going.

Client: (*She continues*) It's heavy.

Therapist: Heavy. That's five.

Give me five more.

Client: It hurts.

It's tired.

Client pauses.

It's burdened.

Therapist: Hurt, tired, burdened, that's eight.

Two more.

Client: Difficult to move sometimes.

Therapist: Difficult to move.

Nine.

And ten?

Client: Weak.

Let the client process her list. After a pause, which facilitates your client's absorbing what she has become aware of about her shoulder, repeat her tenth and ask for one more.

Therapist: Weak is ten.

Great, now I want you to give me just one more.

Give me an eleventh description of your shoulder.

Client: It wants me to slow down.

It is this eleventh description that is the most significant item that needs exploring.

Therapist: (*Repeat back her full eleventh description*)

It wants you to slow down.

Tell me more…

From here, help your client explore what her body wants her to be aware of regarding her shoulder and specifically that it wants her to slow down.

SAFE SPACE CONVERSATION TECHNIQUE

Unlike the other techniques presented in this book, the Safe Space Conversation technique does not focus on your client's body. This technique is helpful to use when your client wants to have a conversation with someone about a past event or future situation, but is reticent or not able to speak directly with that person. This technique is useful when your client has something that needs to be resolved, some unfinished business. By providing your client with the opportunity to have questions answered by another or the ability to tell someone something, healing can occur at a cellular level.

There is a broad range of applications for this technique. Here are some ways that clients use it:

- to tell someone how they feel/felt
- to ask/inquire into why someone did/did not do something
- to talk with someone about a potentially unpleasant future encounter/event/conversation/meeting
- to want someone to know something
- to have a conversation with someone who is deceased, not around, or not able to communicate with the client

- to have a conversation with someone he does not want to see in person, but needs to talk with

There are six components to this technique: the location of the safe space, your client, the other person, the support person (this is optional), talking-stick rules, and the conversation itself.

A safe space

Once your client has identified the situation she wants to address and knows with whom she wants to talk, have your client visualize a comfortable safe space in which the conversation will take place.

1. Have your client visualize a safe space

    - real or imagined
    - knows, has been to, or knows of

2. Have her picture or place herself there.

3. Say, "Tell me when you are there."

    Once she has indicated that she is at her safe space, have your client get a good sense of her surroundings. Have her fully describe the place to you. Ask her to describe her surroundings to help her fully embody where she is. This helps her place herself there. Remember to ask questions using her processing languages, if you know them.

4. Say, "Describe your safe space to me."

5. Have your client get a really good sense of her environment and describe it.

    - (If outside) What season is it?
    - Is it sunny?
    - What is the temperature?
    - Is it breezy?
    - (If inside) Which room in the house is she in?
    - What furniture is there?
    - Are there windows?
    - What is she wearing?
    - Where is she sitting?

Support person

Depending upon the situation, your client may want someone there for support.[1] Sometimes this is helpful so she does not feel alone. Sometimes she may want someone there to speak as a surrogate for her. This support person can be real or imagined, alive or dead. It may be a parent, other family member, or friend. Depending upon your client's beliefs, she may want to invite a guide or angel or other helpful entity to be present with her. Initially, if she does not want anyone with her, inform your client that she can invite a support person to join her at any time.

6. Ask, "Is there anyone you want there with you for support?"

   Inform the client that this support person may be real, alive, passed on, imaginary, a guide, parent, friend, or guardian angel. Be careful that you know her beliefs regarding guides and angels, etc.

   If the client indicates that she does not want a support person, tell her she can always ask for assistance to come in at any time.

The other person

Find out who your client wants to talk with, as well as the general subject matter. As the session progresses, the subject matter may change or shift. This is normal and acceptable. Sometimes what your client actually needs to resolve is slightly different from her original intention.

7. Once the safe space is described and a chosen support person is present, invite in the person with whom your client will converse.
   Say, "Invite [chosen person's name] to come in and have a seat."

8. Have your client describe the features of this person:

   • hair and eye color

   • clothing

   • where the other person is seated

   By having your client describe the person with whom she will be talking, you help her get a full sense of the person. This helps your client have a deeper awareness of the experience. Occasionally, I have had a client who thought that she wanted to talk with one person, but when she tried to get a good sense of that person, the person with whom she originally started talking changed into a different person. Your client may discover that the original person with whom she began the conversation was not,

---

1 This person is different from a guardian angel, as discussed in chapter 8, "Word Choice." The guardian angel supplies information or intercedes for your client. The support person in a Safe Space Conversation is there to lend emotional support, rather than supplying information.

ultimately, the person with whom she needed to communicate to resolve her situation.
If this happens, assure her this is okay and help her shift her conversation to the other
person.

Talking-stick rules

The next step is to explain the rules for the conversation. This technique uses
what are referred to as talking-stick rules. Simply, one person talks at a time,
starting with your client, while the other person listens. You always start and
end with your client speaking, since the session is about her. Your client has the
opportunity to say and ask anything and everything that she wants to know from
the other person. While your client is talking, the other person is listening fully
and completely. I describe to my client that the other person will be listening with
ears wide open, implying that the person will be paying complete attention.

9. Say, "You will go first. You get to say or tell the other person whatever
    you want or to ask any questions of them.

    "While you are speaking, the other person will quietly be listening with
    open ears and full attention. He [or she] won't say or respond until you are
    finished speaking. Then, it is the other person's turn to speak, respond, and
    reply while you are quietly listening with open ears.

    "When the other person is done speaking, you will get a chance to respond,
    answering any questions of his [or hers], replying to anything he [or she]
    has said. You may give him [or her] additional comments as you choose.

    "You will go back and forth until you are both done."

The conversation

Your client can talk aloud or silently to herself. If she speaks the conversation
out loud, it helps her energetically to connect deeper with the situation and
conversation. Having your client talk out loud also prevents her from drifting
off to sleep. It prevents her from avoiding the conversation, and it prevents her
from changing what she thinks she wants to say. All that being said, sometimes
the situation is tender or a bit private or might even be perceived by the client
as embarrassing, so she might prefer to speak this silently. If she is conversing
silently, have her indicate when she is finished with each section. As long as
she stays on track and lets you know when each section is complete, it is fine to
continue silently.

If she chooses to have this conversation quietly, make sure you are paying
attention to your Indicator Compass. If your client gets stuck, goes off track,

or starts zoning out, her body will indicate this by signaling your Indicator Compass.

When your client is done, it is the other person's turn. The other person gets a chance to respond to any questions that were asked and to ask any of his or her own. Now is the other person's turn to reply to anything that your client spoke. The other person also has the opportunity to tell your client anything he or she wants to communicate.

Initially, some clients have a difficult time trusting how and what they think the other person might respond. I encourage them to speak whatever comes immediately to mind. Sometimes I say, "What would George say if he were sitting there in front of you?"

As the conversation happens, have your client speak in first person. This is especially important when she is talking with the other person. If your client says, "I want to tell George that I really don't understand why he…," have her shift her dialogue so she is speaking directly to George. The conversation needs to happen between your client and George, not between your client and you: "George, I really don't understand why you…" Having your client speak in first person and directly to the other person helps her to embody the session more fully.

Some clients will use their own voice out loud for both sides of the conversation. It is not unusual for the sound of your client's voice to change as the other person speaks: "Carol, I'm sorry that you don't understand why I…" Other clients will report what the other person has told them: "He is telling me that he is sorry that I don't understand why…" Either way is acceptable. The important point is to have your client not censor or filter anything that the other person is communicating to her.

Next round

After the first round, your client can respond with any answers to questions, ask more questions, or give further comments. This is done back and forth, one person talking at a time, until your client (and the person with whom she is conversing) is finished. The conversation is complete when your client has asked and said all that she needs to communicate. Some conversations will be brief, with each person only speaking two or three times. Other conversations can be extensive, going back and forth numerous times. An answer resolving your client's situation is often received, but this is not a necessary outcome. Sometimes, your client may gain information that provides her with an insight into the situation with which she might need to do additional work at a later time.

The therapist's role

As a therapist, your role is to be the observer. Occasionally, you may need to be a moderator to ensure that the talking-stick rules are followed. Be sure that you do not interject your thoughts as to what your client should or should not say to the other person or how to interpret the conversation. Before this part of the session, your client may have revealed that she wants to say something in particular. This may have changed, so if you do feel compelled to interject "Do you want to tell him…?" make sure you use lots of Wiggle Words as you do so, giving your client permission to change or alter anything that you say.

Starting the conversation

At this point, your client has described her safe space and identified the topic of the conversation. All parties involved are present: your client, her support person (if desired), and the person with whom she will talk. Everyone knows the talking-stick rules. Now, it is time to begin the conversation.

10.   You might say,

"So, go ahead. Tell him what you would like to know. Ask what you would like to ask, while he patiently listens with open ears."

If your client has opted to speak quietly within herself, you should add,

"Let me know when you are done."

11.   When your client indicates that she is finished, you should say something like,

"Now it's his turn. What would he like to say?"

and add, if she is speaking inwardly,

"Let me know when he is done."

Sometimes the client feels silly, unsure, or stupid or as if she is fabricating the reply. If she makes a comment of this nature, assure her that it is normal to feel silly and just to go with it. If she is still unsure about the reply, ask her to feel the answer deep down inside, coming from her intuition: "If he had just heard your question, thoughts, etc., what would he say in response? Just go with it." Help her to not second-guess herself. Using your Indicator Compass, help your client trust her intuition by affirming accuracy or significance when your indicator designates something as being on track.

12.   Go back and forth until all participants are done with the conversation. Remember that your client has the last word. Make sure that your client has asked and said all she needs to:

"Is there anything else you would like to say?"

When she indicates that she is completely finished, say,

"Thank him [the person she has been speaking to] for coming and speaking with you and show him the way out."

13.   Afterward, I allow some quiet time for my client to process and integrate what occurred during the conversation. Eventually, I inquire "Thoughts, comments, questions?" to give her the invitation to say whatever she would like about the session.

Safe Space Conversation, abbreviated technique

1.   Find out with whom your client wants to talk and the general subject matter.

   Both the subject and conversation may change or shift as the session progresses. This is normal and acceptable.

2.   Have your client visualize a safe space that:

   • is real or imagined

   • she knows, has been to, or knows of

   • she can picture or put herself there

3.   Say, "Tell me when you are there."

4.   Say, "Describe your safe space to me."

   This helps her fully to embody and place herself there.

5.   Have the client get a really good sense of her environment and describe it.

   • (If outside) What season is it?

   • Is it sunny?

   • What is the temperature?

   • Is it breezy?

   • (If inside) Which room in the house is she in?

   • What furniture is there?

   • Are there windows?

   • What is she wearing?

   • Where is she sitting?

6. Ask, "Is there anyone you want there with you for support?"

   Inform the client that this support person may be real, alive, passed on, imaginary, a guide, parent, friend, or guardian angel. Be careful that you know her beliefs regarding guides and angels, etc.

   If the client indicates that she does not want a support person, tell her she can always ask for assistance to come in at any time.

7. Say, "Invite [name of person with whom she will converse] to come in and have a seat."

8. Have your client describe the features of this person:

   • hair and eye color

   • clothing

   • where he is seated

   By having your client describe the person with whom she will be talking, you help her get a full sense of the person.

9. Explain how the conversation will happen, using talking-stick rules:

   "You will go first. You get to say and or tell him whatever you want or to ask any questions.

   "While you are speaking, he will quietly be listening with open ears and full attention. He won't say or respond until you are done. Then it is his turn to speak, respond, and reply while you are quietly listening with open ears. [This is the talking-stick rule.]

   "When he is done, you will get a chance to respond, answering any questions of his, replying to anything he has said. You may tell him additional things if you choose.

   "You will go back and forth until you are done.

   "So, go ahead. Tell him what you would like to know; ask what you would like to ask, while he patiently listens with open ears."

   If the client is speaking quietly, in her head, say, "Let me know when you are done."

   "Now it's his turn. What would he like to say?"

   "Let me know when he is done."

   Go back and forth until done.

   "Anything else you would like to say?"

When your client is finished, say, "Thank him for coming and speaking with you and show him the way out."

"So…thoughts, comments, questions?"

Sonja's story

What happens in these sessions can be quite profound. A simple example is Sonja's session. Sonja was 24 years old and a single mother of a three-year-old son. Her father lived in a city three hours away from her. He had seen his grandson only a couple of times, and, even though he lived relatively nearby, he was never interested in visiting Sonja and his grandson. Sonja was sad about this and about the fact that her father had never told her that he loved her. For Sonja's session, she wanted to talk with her father and find out why he did not want to see them. She also wanted to know why he did not tell her that he loved her when they spoke on the phone.

We had Sonja find her safe space and invite her father in. She described what her father looked like and the clothes he wore. She started by telling him how it hurt her that he did not want to see her and her son. The conversation continued with their discussing how she would like him to visit and see his grandson. In the session, he explained to her that he had been uncertain about some things in his own life and that he felt awkward telling her that he loved her. Some of his last words to her during her safe-space conversation were "Sonja, I love you."

Sonja left my office with a smile on her face and a sense of being cared for by her father, even though she thought it was unlikely that anything with her father would change.

Three weeks later, Sonja arrived for her next appointment. She told me that about a week after her session, her father had called. Without her telling him anything about the session, he told her, "I love you"—and he wanted to make arrangements to see his grandson and her.

11 Meet the Twins

RESISTANCE VERSUS

PROTECTION AND THEIR

ROLE IN HEALING

RESISTANCE

Chapter 6, "Dialoguing," discussed many reasons why your client may not want to dialogue. Additionally, information was presented about why a client might not know how to dialogue. You now have the fundamental principles of working with what is commonly referred to as "resistance": your client feels unsafe, fears, or does not know how to get in touch with, what is going on in her body, is blocking, and becomes disconnected.

The online *American Heritage Dictionary* defines *resistance* as:

1. the act or an instance of resisting or the capacity to resist

2. a force that tends to oppose or retard motion

3. a process in which the ego opposes the conscious recall of anxiety-producing experiences

4.　a.　the capacity of an organism to defend itself against a disease
　　b.　the capacity of an organism or a tissue to withstand the effects of a harmful environmental agent

For the sake of conversation, *resistance* shall be defined here as a force or process that has the ability to oppose progress, especially when the force perceives the changes as being detrimental to itself, rather than perceiving them as being beneficial to its host.

That is a mouthful, I admit! Let us break it down. What is often considered as resistance is a force or process that has resided in a host, your client's body. I know that this makes it seem already as if resistance is a living organism that has a mind of its own. Yes, that is what it wants your client and you to believe. Therefore, in this chapter, I will personify Resistance (capital *R*) and its twin, Protection (capital *P*). Resistance will oppose your client's healing because it perceives changes and awarenesses as detrimental to itself. Resistance does not care about your client and what is best for him. Resistance is only interested in doing its job and whatever is necessary to maintain self-preservation. The force of Resistance can be so strong that it will prevent any change to its environment, your client's body. It will do this through procrastination, delays, or even self-destructive and self-sabotaging acts. How often have you heard from a client, "I know I should exercise/eat right/ forgive my brother, etc., but I just can't seem to do it. I don't know what is wrong with me."

Resistance is only interested in doing its job. At an earlier time, Resistance was assigned a job or responsibility by your client. It may have been your client's conscious awareness or it may have been your client's subconscious. Regardless, Resistance has a job to do, and it will not stop until it is fully informed that the job is no longer necessary and is given further instructions.

"Wait a minute! What do you mean I don't have a job anymore?" I can hear Resistance bellowing.

Yes, this is where your client needs to educate and negotiate with Resistance about what is currently true as opposed to what happened in the past. But before you go there, you need to know a little about Resistance's twin.

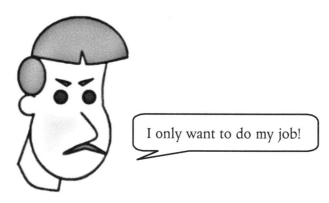

PROTECTION

Meet Resistance's twin: Protection. Protection has been with you since before you were born. Protection knows everything about you. Well, almost. Protection knows more than enough about you and the world to keep you safe. It is hard-wired with a list of responsibilities, even before you are born. Protection's only purpose and responsibility in life is to keep you safe.

Do you remember the first time you put your hand on a hot stove? Your mother may have been standing right there and shouted at you "No! That's hot! Don't touch!" as she grabbed your hand away from the stove. She was being Protection's surrogate for the moment. Parents are good at doing that. Even if no one was around to pull your hand off the hot stove, Protection was there. With a quick recoiling of your hand and arm, Protection would have made you pull your hand away from the heat before you burned yourself too badly. That is Protection's job—keeping you safe. And that is fortunate since protective parents are not always around.

How about that snake you saw slinking down the path? What did you do? Did you freeze? Protection made you do it. When you and Protection identified it as a harmless, nonpoisonous garter snake, then protection allowed you to take a deep breath and relax. Had it been poisonous, however, Protection would have kept you on heightened alert until you were quietly able to get away.

Protection's job varies from person to person. If you are allergic to bees, then Protection will keep a good look out for any honey bees feeding in the clover tucked in the grass. If you are not allergic to bees, then it would be rather pointless and silly for Protection to make you tip toe through the clover. Okay, I know you do not want to step on a bee purposefully, but Protection will not waste its precious time and energy doing everything for you. Caution is your job.

Sometimes, through on-the-job experience, Protection is assigned a job by your conscious or subconscious awareness. Often this job assignment comes as a result of an accident, illness, or trauma. This occurred when your body was hurt or experienced something very unpleasant; it does not want to have this experience again. For example, an extreme dislike of spicy foods can be the result of Protection's kicking into action after you suffered a severe reaction.

One night you might have gone to a friend's house for dinner, and she served something that tasted so delicious that you did not pay attention to the ingredients. As you took a delightfully large bite, you ate a big piece of hot pepper. What you did not realize was that it was a very, very hot pepper, and it burned your tongue, your mouth, and all the way down to your stomach. You can laugh now, but it was not funny at the time you grabbed for something to cool things down. Actually, at that moment of looking for the fire extinguisher, your body already told Protection to make sure that you avoid spicy-looking food to prevent future internal wildfires.

THE TWINS GET CONFUSED

Let me tell you about a client of mine, Corey. Corey attended a university in a very safe city. The university campus was also considered very safe. One evening, Corey walked by herself in the dark. Unfortunately, she was attacked, right there on campus. From then on, Protection would make her startle at every little noise she heard. Protection made her jump even in her own house, even in broad day light, even when she knew that the noise was her cat in the next room playing with a toy. Corey had a difficult time sleeping because her body was constantly jumping as Protection had her on a heightened state of alertness. This heightened state of alertness was especially important when she was alone in the dark in places where she had no control. However, this jumpiness was actually harming her by preventing her from getting rest at night. It was not beneficial, and she was unable to relax or study or enjoy life.

If you are allergic to bees, Protection is helpful. If you are near hot things that could burn you, Protection is helpful. If you eat spicy food, Protection may need to make you cautious. If you are around snakes, Protection may or may not be necessary. During the night in strange places, Protection walked with Corey, along with the mace spray, helping to keep her safe. But who makes her jumpy during the day or in her own home? Protection? Or Protection's twin, Resistance? It was not Protection—it was Resistance.

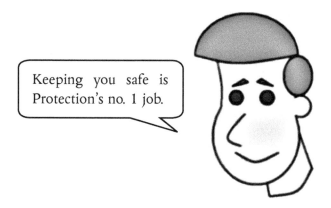

Protection and Resistance are, as the saying goes, different sides of the same coin. On one side, Protection is beneficial and helpful and wanted. When its job is no longer necessary or no longer beneficial and it continues to act, however, it becomes Resistance. Like a spinning or tossed-up coin, sometimes it is difficult to figure out which is which. They really are the same force; one is desired and helpful, while the other often impedes progress and drains energy.

Here are a few more important details about Protection and Resistance. Resistance arises when something is scary or painful for your client. Remember that this is actually a protective mechanism that the client's body has put in place to keep him safe. Feelings that are scary or painful or memories of an unpleasant past can automatically trigger a sense of being unsafe, which activates the protective mechanism.

When your client becomes aware of Resistance, he needs to explore its purpose. Occasionally, it will not be necessary for your client to know what Resistance's job was or how it got there. More often than not, however, a client finds it helpful to have those details. Determining Resistance's purpose gives your client information as to whether its job is still beneficial, even to the smallest degree. Sometimes Resistance has a message for your clients, so again help him determine the message from Resistance. It is interesting what happens when Resistance is able to deliver its message. Quite often, that is sufficient to allow it to disappear. Its job is done, its message is delivered, and it can disperse.

Resistance is actually an old protective mechanism that is no longer needed anymore or is no longer beneficial. And this is how I like to help a client think about it—something that is no longer needed. When a client can come to the awareness and realization that something is no longer beneficial or needed, then it is much easier for him to allow his body to release it.

It is similar to keeping an old beat-up frying pan around the kitchen when you have a nice gourmet-quality skillet available to do the same job. When you realize, "Oh, yeah, I don't need to keep the old one any longer. It's all worn out, and the handle is almost falling off," it is a lot easier to recycle it. When you think that you still need it, that you do not have anything else to do the work, then you are more likely to be resistant to disposing of it. Corey's body did not want to let go of the jumpiness and alertness because Protection/Resistance did not know that it no longer needed to be "on duty" all the time.

WORKING WITH THE COIN

Go back to the beginning of this chapter and the definition of the word *resistance*: a force or process that has the ability to oppose progress, especially when the force perceives the changes as being detrimental to itself, rather than perceiving them as being beneficial to its host. Let us examine more about how to work with that force, Resistance, that perceives changes as being detrimental.

Once you told yourself that you had a wonderful skillet to use in the kitchen rather than the dented frying pan, it was easy to relinquish the old one. It would be nice if the situation were that smooth with getting rid of Resistance. Sometimes all that needs to happen is for your client to realize that Protection has transformed into Resistance. She needs to realize the transformation and let Resistance know that the old protective mechanism is no longer necessary. Resistance may put up a fight. It may dig its heels in and protest, "But what about...?" Simply having your client reassure Resistance that it is okay and informing it that the situation has changed may be enough for it to be willing to go away.

Sometimes Resistance likes to make your client believe that it will die if it stops doing its job. No one likes to look mortality in the face, not even Resistance. If Resistance believes it will die, it will do all that it can to prevent this from happening. It will do everything it can to hang on and keep doing its job, even if the job is no longer relevant or necessary. This is where sitting down at the negotiating table is necessary. You begin to facilitate change by having your client educate Resistance about the facts and about the future.

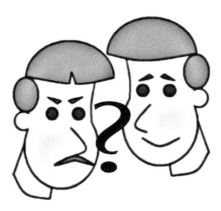

Facts to educate Resistance include:

- what the past situation was that necessitated the protective mechanism

- what changed so that the protective mechanism is no longer necessary

- what will happen to the host body (your client) that Resistance is living in if Resistance continues doing what it has been. (Your client will often have an awareness that something detrimental could happen to her if Resistance continues to stay.)

- what could happen beneficially for the host body (your client) if Resistance resigns and leaves

Once Resistance has been informed by your client of the entire situation, then it is easier to work with this force. If Resistance is not willing to disappear completely and leave, then some job negotiating is necessary. Sometimes a small part of

Resistance is needed because your client may not feel comfortable if her safety blanket is gone entirely. Here are a couple of analogies that I like to use.

One is "eat one pea at a time." This is about focusing on a small part of the situation at a time, not looking at the huge pile of peas, but just looking at a few of them. When those few are gone, then work with the next little bit of Resistance. Have your client continue to work bit by bit to release Resistance until it is gone.

Another way to work with it is to have Resistance shrink in size. Quite often when a client starts describing this force, he realizes that Resistance takes up a lot of space and a lot of energy. When he is able to shrink Resistance (toss it in the dryer, put it in a zapping machine, put it out to dry like a grape shrinking into a raisin—let him use his imagination), then it often loses its strength and loosens its hold on his body. If a small part of Resistance is still necessary for whatever reason, shrinking it and having it be in an innocuous place so that it does not get in the way of everyday life is a wonderful way to negotiate with it.

Then there is the worst-case scenario. This situation might sound very serious and possibly scary or even life-threatening, and it could possibly be true for your client if Resistance does not give up its job. One scenario played out like this:

> *Therapist*: I'd like you take a moment and get a good sense of that area of your body that has been getting your attention [referring to Resistance]. Let me know when you have a good sense of it.
>
> *Client*: Yup.
>
> *Therapist*: Okay, now that you have a good sense of it I'd like you to take a moment and let your body make you aware of what could happen if this stayed in your body. What is the worst thing that could happen?
>
> *Client*: (*Pause*)
>
> *Therapist*: Let me know when you have a sense of it.
>
> *Client*: Yup.
>
> *Therapist*: What are you aware of that is the worst thing that could happen if this [Resistance] stayed with you?
>
> *Client*: I'd get sick...
>
>   [or]
>
> I'd get cancer...
>
>   [or]
>
> I'd never get well...
>
>   [or]
>
> I won't have any energy...

Therapist: And what would happen to it [Resistance]?

Client: It would…

> *Often what would happen to Resistance is the same or worse as would happen to your client.*

Therapist: What would you like to do now that you are aware that the worst thing that could happen is _____ [repeat back what client told you] and _____ would happen to Resistance?

Client: I want to _____ (*responds accordingly*).

Therapist: (*Continues to facilitate the session according to client's directive.*)

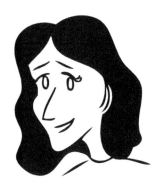

Thanks for doing a great job. We're all done. Everyone can go home now and relax.

BODYGUARD JOB REASSIGNMENT TECHNIQUE

The Bodyguard Job Reassignment technique is also known as reassigning Resistance to a new job position. It is especially helpful with situations like Corey's as described above. She gave her bodyguard a new job. Here is how the dialoguing went:

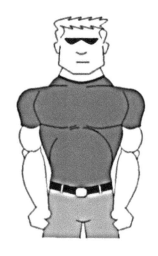

> *Therapist* (me): So you've identified a part of you that makes you edgy, jumpy, and on alert all the time. You have told me that you don't need this anymore and would like to get rid of it. Am I correct?
>
> *Client* (Corey): Yes, that's right, but I don't know if I'm ready to let all of it go yet. It feels as if I need to keep some of it around.
>
> *Therapist*: Okay. So, instead of having it around all the time, what if you gave it a job reassignment?

Client: Okay...

Therapist: For example, and you are welcome to use or change any of this, instead of having a bodyguard protecting you 24/7/365, walking around hovering over you all the time, what if you gave that bodyguard a job reassignment to a night watchman? He could have a chair and sit at a desk with lots of monitors to watch and make sure you are safe. He'd have a telephone to call for back-up. And he could have a radio if he needed to alert you about anything. And, if necessary, there could even be a big panic button he could press if he needs to get your immediate attention. But most of the time he could just sit there and kick back and eat donuts. How does that sound?

Client: That sounds good. I'd actually like him to _____.

> *Encourage client to make any changes to fit her purposes and needs. Or if she has a different idea completely, use it.*

Therapist: Okay, what I'd like you to do now is get a good sense of that part of you that has been your bodyguard. Let me know what you are aware of.

Client: Yup.

Therapist: Okay, what is your bodyguard's name?

Client: Bob.

Therapist: Okay, please say "Hi" to Bob, and let him know the situation. He's been working very hard, working 24/7/365 for _____ [specify amount of time]. He's been doing a really good job. [I only say this if I know he has been doing a good job based on what my client has told me.] And he's been making you feel _____ [however Resistance has made the client feel— tired, sick, unhappy, etc.]. Let him know that he doesn't have to work so hard anymore because the situation has changed and he is going to get a new and easier job. Let him know that he can now be a night watchman. Starting now.

Client: (*Either quietly to herself or out loud tells Bob all this information and then acknowledges when this has happened.*)

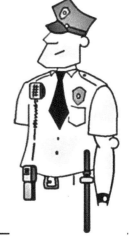

Therapist: Okay. How are you doing, _____ [client's name]?

Client: (*Responds accordingly.*)

Therapist: How is Bob?

Client: (*Responds accordingly.*)

Therapist: Anything else you two need or want to tell each other?

Client: (*Responds accordingly.*)

Therapist: (*Wraps up the dialoguing section.*)

Sometimes Bob the Bodyguard may not want to accept his reassignment for fear that he will not be able to act fast enough or get my client's attention. Some negotiations need to be done when my client wants to reassign the bodyguard, but there is reluctance on the bodyguard's behalf. One of the most effective ways to achieve this resolution is to let the bodyguard know that he can sit in front of a panel of television monitors that constantly watch my client. There is also a big, red panic button that he, as the night watchman, can press if he needs to get her attention quickly.

Sometimes it is necessary to include additional communication tools, such as a special phone line or agreed-upon words or phrases, to assure clear communication. Negotiations may require a couple of agreed-upon indicators for different levels of danger. A general warning may require a whisper in the client's ear: "Be careful." When the situation seems a little more dangerous, there might be a stronger statement: "Keep your wits about you." And extreme situations might dictate that there be a shouting of "Danger! Stop!" Depending upon your client, the line of communication may need to be felt kinesthetically. This results in the client's experiencing a particular sensation in a benign manner, such as tingling in the left pinky finger or feeling as if someone were tapping on her shoulder.

Other suggestions I offer a client to help release Resistance include trying the situation out in the office, vacuuming Resistance out of his body, putting it in the garbage can, and giving it an eviction notice. If my client is not sure about letting go of Resistance entirely, I offer the idea that he try it in the office. I tell him something like the following: "Give it a try while you are here, during this session. If you want to allow your body to let go fully of Resistance, you can try it out here. You can get a sense of how it is for you here. If you want to pick it up at the door when you leave, you can. Otherwise…" and I just let my voice trail off while he quietly fills in the rest of my sentence.

Quite often, the client does decide to try it. We then go about helping his body release Resistance in whatever manner works for him. In all the years that I have been doing this, I have not had someone pick it up on his way out. He is quite happy to be leaving a few pounds lighter.

And when your client is really ready to get completely rid of Resistance but it is being stubborn, then it might be necessary to give it an eviction notice. Let your client's imagination run wild with ideas about how to help his body release Resistance.

These analogies are lots of fun for clients to work with, but they are not always necessary or appropriate. Quiet often, your client will be able easily and effortlessly to have Resistance dissolve or melt away or drift out of his body, just by becoming aware of it and recognizing it for what it is and for what it is not. Please respect this, and do not force your clients into working any harder than is necessary.

LOOKING AT THE HEAD OF THE COIN

When you work with a client and what seems to be Resistance has come up, you need to have your client make sure that it is not needed any more. You and your client need to honor this protection mechanism if part of her believes that this protection mechanism is still necessary. Honor it if it would be detrimental to your client for your client to release this protection mechanism. Bodies have an innate knowing that the conscious mind sometimes cannot comprehend. If in doubt, like the situation with the snake, respect it and leave it alone. If your client wants more help with the protection mechanisms, refer her on to someone more experienced with this type of situation.

Which twin: Protection or Resistance?

As previously mentioned but worth repeating again, make sure you hold a safe space, keep yourself centered and grounded, and have no judgments or preconceived notions about the situation. These techniques of working to resolve Resistance build upon the fundamentals that have been previously discussed. If you are not reading these chapters in sequential order, please make sure you read the material that corresponds to these different sections.

1. Bring your client's awareness into her body.

    If there is difficulty doing this, refer to chapter 6, "Dialoguing," and the technique "How to Get Started" discussed in chapter 10, "Getting Started."

2. Give your client permission to:

    • feel

    • be there

    If necessary do the Permission technique with her, as described in chapter 10, "Getting Started."

3. Protection: Identify which category Protection falls into:

    • current and helpful

    • learned

    • learned and helpful in past

- learned and helpful currently
- irrelevant

   If Protection is not currently helpful or beneficial and is no longer necessary, then continue helping your client identify it. It is now considered Resistance or a gremlin.

4. As described earlier, work with Resistance or a gremlin:

    - identify it
    - identify its purpose
    - identify the message Resistance or the gremlin has

5. Have your client determine if Resistance is still needed. Have your client determine if any of it is worth keeping. Should she keep some of it or get rid of it all?

6. What does your client want to do with it? As described previously in this chapter, ask your client what she wants to do with Resistance. Below are some ways to help your client decide:

    - Say, "Let me know if you need any help or would like a suggestion."
    - Offer a variety of things other clients have done in the past. Use Wiggle Words when offering suggestions so that your client is empowered to make the situation her own.
    - Does she want to give Resistance an eviction notice?
    - Does she want to negotiate with Resistance?
    - Does she want to offer Resistance a job reassignment: from being a bodyguard (24/7/365 on duty) to being a night watchman?

Free trip to Hawaii

With all that you have learned thus far, help your client identify Resistance, determine what Resistance wants and is willing to do, and what your client wants to do with Resistance. Sometimes Resistance gets in the way because that is what it likes to do and knows how to do well. Sometimes it just wants to muck things up and slow down your client's healing process.

This sometimes shows up as Brain talking and trying to tell your client stuff, rather than your client being able to communicate clearly and directly with a specific area of his body. One of the best ways to deal with this is to give Brain a one-way ticket to Hawaii for a vacation.

   Therapist: Is that Body or Brain speaking?

(Pay attention to your Indicator Compass as your client responds.)

Client: Ummm. Body? I'm not sure.

Therapist: It sounds to me, and correct me if I'm wrong, that Brain is doing the talking.

Any hesitation is an indication that it is Brain, not Body. Pay attention to your Indicator Compass.

Client: Yeah, I guess you're right.

Therapist: Let's do this. If it's all right with you, let's have you give Brain a pina colada [or mai tai or rum runner—your choice; I happen to like pina coladas] and a one-way ticket to Hawaii or somewhere warm. Let Brain go on a vacation, while you and Body do some work here. [By this time, the client is laughing or trying not to.] When we're done, we'll send it a ticket so it can come back. How does that sound to you?

Client: Sounds good!

What is this really about? What you have actually just told your client's subconscious is that you are paying attention and that you did notice that his brain started talking rather than letting his body communicate with him. "Oops!" It got caught. Once caught in the act, Brain knows that it might as well go on vacation because it will have a difficult time sneaking past your alertness.

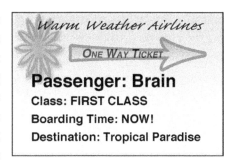

Warm Weather Airlines

ONE WAY TICKET

Passenger: Brain
Class: FIRST CLASS
Boarding Time: NOW!
Destination: Tropical Paradise

Monsters

All this talk about Resistance and gremlins and messages brings to mind a wonderful book. A teacher of mine told the class one day that he lends it out to clients. I was familiar with the book because I had it as a child, but it was not until I read it again that I realized how it applied to my clients who are struggling with Resistance.

Find a copy of the Sesame Street book *The Monster at the End of This Book* (by Jon Stone). It features the blue monster, Grover. Read it to a child and get into Grover's character. When you are done with the book, you will have heard multiple times that if you keep going, you will get to the end of the book and have to face a nasty monster. Grover warns you not to turn the pages; he even tries his best efforts to block you from doing so by tying them, nailing them, and building a brick wall. Similarly, quite often a client is afraid to "go there" or open the closet door or talk with the "nasty" part of herself for fear of what she might find.

At the end of the book, due to your strength and perseverance, you learn, much to Grover's embarrassment, that the monster is just furry, lovable Grover himself.

Now a bit about other monsters. Alien movies are not what they used to be because the alien monster is revealed quite early in the movie, so it leaves you with nothing to be scared of. Movies like *The Creature from the Black Lagoon* or the original *Alien* or more recently in the 1990s the movie *Signs* have kept the monster scary and scary throughout the entire movie. They do this by showing you the havoc the monster is causing and only giving you a teensy bit of information about the creature. As the movie progresses, you learn more a little bit at a time about the creature. This continues until right at the end when the monster is revealed. Because you and the hero/heroine now know all about the monster creature, you also know how to deal with it. You know how to destroy it.

It is the same with your client. Initially, to look at Resistance and gremlins can be very scary and off-putting. But when your client is able to gather information bit by bit, she is able to get a better picture of it. She is able to get a better sense and look at the actual situation. Your client soon realizes that her "creature" has been trying to get her attention or protect her in some manner. When your client is able to identify her "creature" for what it really is, the scariness disappears, and awareness and realizations can occur. Remember that this is the purpose and goal of SomaCentric Dialoguing—helping your client become more aware of what is happening in her body so that she can take better care of herself.

12 Gems and Nuances

The expression "little things make a difference" holds true in SomaCentric Dialoguing. What transforms a science into an art form is quite often the nuances that are developed and applied. In this chapter, you will explore differences that help facilitate a session and make it smoother. Additionally, you will learn about how to apply nuances to the SomaCentric Dialoguing skills you have been learning. This chapter also includes what I consider to be gems, little concepts that can easily be used, sometimes with great impact.

WHY HANDS ON?

After her session, Meg told me how important it was for her that my hands were in contact with her body while we were SomaCentric Dialoguing. She said that it made the dialoguing more effective. Putting hands on your client's body helps:

- your client to stay connected to her body sensations in an easier and deeper manner

- you pay attention to your Indicator Compass by listening to your client's tissues under your hands and to what is going on

- ground your client with the process that she is experiencing

- nonverbally communicate to your client that you are paying attention

Putting your hands on your client lets her know that you are there with her, lets her know on a nonverbal level that she is not alone. Often a client believes that she is alone in her situation and experience. She believes that she is all by herself and has to do everything on her own. Having your hands on your client sends her a message that you are there with her as a witness and as support. Contact can be as simple as cradling her head or gently resting your hand on her arm or leg. She still has to do all the work by herself, but when her subconscious knows that someone is with her, it helps make things less scary and less overwhelming.

This does not mean that you cannot do SomaCentric Dialoguing effectively without putting your hands on your clients. You can do SomaCentric Dialoguing without utilizing touch, but this requires that you very carefully track your client, making sure she stays on course. If you work with your client in a hands-off manner, make sure you utilize statements and questions that help keep her focused and centered in her body-awarenesses.

"ONE MORE TIME" VERSUS "AND AGAIN"

When a therapist says, "One more time," generally it means only one more time will the client be asked to do something, and then that part is over. When something that is asked of your client seems uncomfortable or unpleasant, it is sometimes a relief for your client to hear you say, "One more time." You have now told him that he is done after this last time. Did you really mean it, though? Or do you catch yourself saying, "One more time," when you actually mean you want him to do something again and again?

Frustration can easily strike when one more time turns into three more "One more times." This frustration can be underlying and not apparent. Your client may build up tension in his body as an unconscious response to repeated "One more times." I strongly suggest that you avoid using the phrase "One more time" unless you really mean it. If you want your client to do something again, simply say, "And again." Mean what you say, and say what you mean.

TIME-CAPSULE CONCEPTS

Time can play an important part in a session. Here you will learn about three different concepts that can impact the session: finding the time, anniversaries, and flash-pan thoughts.

Finding the time

It may be important to determine when the first experience of an emotion or physical complaint occurred. I call this "finding the time." If your client can identify the first time she felt something, she generally will have an easier time identifying the situation that contributed to her current state. When your client is able to identify and resolve the first incidence of the situation, then her body can stop carrying around that energetic signature and begin healing what is happening in the present time.

Here are two examples of this phenomenon. The first I described in chapter 8, "Word Choice," and the second will be explored in chapter 13, "Creating a Session." The first example involves Susan. When we inquired about her first experience of a particular feeling, she initially believed that it was in fifth grade. As she stayed with the feeling, she realized that it was actually third grade, two years earlier. This recognition made a huge difference because the situation that happened in third grade impacted what happened in fifth grade. Susan trusted herself to correct herself and make sure which occurrence was the first time. Sometimes clients will need assistance to do this.

To help your client determine when she experienced something for the first time have her get a good sense of what her body feels like in the current time, right then and there. Then ask her to go back, maybe a year or a couple of years, to determine the first time she experienced the situation. If a client tells you, "Quite a long time," have her clarify this vague statement by asking, "Do you mean five years? Ten years? Twenty?" Make sure to use a question to which she has to come up with the answer.

When she provides you with a time, she might say, "It feels like I'm seventeen." Encourage her to check it out. Get a good sense of the experience at age seventeen and what her body feels like. Ask her to determine if she first experienced the feeling at a younger age and reiterate your instructions that she wants to determine the first time she experienced it: "Make sure, check it out and get a good sense of it. Check out if it was then or when you were any younger. Go back to the first time you felt this." Be aware that the first time she had that experience in her body may have been in a slightly different circumstance than what she currently experiences. Let your client know that this is acceptable. Sometimes she will say something like "It is kind of like when I was sixteen and…" The sense of "kind of like" is going to be a very good starting point.

The second example will be found in the next chapter. You will read about Karen and how something that happened two years prior affected her current life.

Know that it is okay if you do not happen to get the very first incidence. If your client brings something up and your Indicator Compass is working, you will be able to help guide her to the significant situation that her unconscious needs her to work on that day. Sometimes, as was the case with Susan, your client may say that she has worked before on the same situation. Reassure her that her body brings her back to this situation because there is something that still needs to be addressed. If she says that she has already worked on that situation, have her check it out and determine if there is anything else her body wants her to know. Start using the SomaCentric Dialoguing techniques you have learned. If your Indicator Compass is unclear, you could also ask your client to find an earlier time when she experienced something similar, but perhaps (Wiggle Word) differently.

And once the situation in the past is resolved, like the example with Susan, have your client bring forward, from the past to present day, what her body has learned and resolved.

Anniversaries

Often, a client will experience a problem around the time of an anniversary. This anniversary is one when something significant happened. The client determines the significance of the event. For example, it may be the anniversary of an abusive attack, a fight, the death of a loved one, a move, loss of a job, an injury, or a surgery. There are two sessions in this book that illustrate how anniversaries play an important role in healing. The first is the session with Patricia found in chapter 6, "Dialoguing," under the heading "Meet Patricia" and the second is with Karen in the next chapter.

A clue for you, the therapist, that an anniversary may be involved is if a client reports to you that he experiences something at the same time of the year. Quite often, he initially thinks that it might be related to the change in seasons or something weather-related. Sometimes a client believes that it is just a coincidence. I tend to question this because I have observed many sessions that were related to anniversaries. Anniversaries can be very powerful. Sometimes the simple act of your client identifying the connection between an anniversary and his current state can be very therapeutic in and of itself. Remember to allow your client to make the discoveries. You are welcome to help facilitate or cautiously guide him. Use Wiggle Words and own your own statements and observations, keep your prejudices away, and empower your client to change anything that does not work for him.

March 1968

S	M	T	W	Th	F	S
					1	2
3	4	5	6	7	8	9
10	11	12	13	14	15	16
17	18	19	20	21	22	23
24	25	26	27	28	29	30
31						

Flash-pan thoughts

The third time-capsule concept is about split-second awarenesses. Like the flash-pan of an antique rifle, things can go "Bang!" quickly, and these are to be acknowledged and honored. When you work with a client and use various techniques, your client should be giving you her immediate responses. She should give you her gut reaction. These are what I call "flash-pan thoughts." These are the images and thoughts that immediately come to mind without analysis. There is an expression, "Analysis leads to paralysis." This is especially true when it comes to SomaCentric Dialoguing.

Encourage your client to trust her first instinct, to go with her gut reaction, to listen to her intuition. As a therapist, trust your first responses when you work with clients and pay attention to your Indicator Compass. These first reactions and responses are highly valid. Learn to trust them. When your client starts to second guess or doubt or tries to rationalize a response, she is drawn out of her body-awareness and up into her head. SomaCentric Dialoguing is about helping your client tune in with what is going on in her body and becoming aware of what her body wants her to know. Analyzing and rationalizing answers are not SomaCentric Dialoguing. Trusting those first impressions is SomaCentric Dialoguing. It may take a little practice, and you may need to reassure your doubting-Thomas client. Once your client gets the hang of SomaCentric Dialoguing, she will learn to trust her first reactions more easily.

There is a wonderful book called *Blink* about the validity of trusting first responses. The author, Malcolm Gladwell, does a superb job explaining why and how decisions made in the blink of an eye are to be trusted. I encourage you to pick it up and read it. It will help strengthen your own trust with what you are tuning in to and thus will help your clients.

TONE/INFLECTION/PACING—USING YOUR VOICE

Along with what is said, the tone, inflection, and pacing of what is spoken are important. There are many books that talk about how tone and inflection can be used to convey different messages, so I will not delve into the details. I will remind you that you need to make sure that your tone and inflection are not judgmental, leading, or condescending to your client. Review chapter 8, "Word Choice," for suggestions on how to avoid judgment and leading statements or questions.

Regarding pacing, ask your questions or make statements and observations in a slow, relaxed manner. I do not mean you should use a hypnotic, slow, flat, monotone voice. Just do not rush the situation. Give your client time to react and respond. Remember that SomaCentric Dialoguing is multifaceted. For your client, there are many different things going on during a session. Give him an opportunity to process what is happening within himself. Ask one question at a time, and give him ample time to respond fully.

Sometimes you may have an entire train of thought to explore and a list of possible questions to ask. Avoid getting ahead of yourself and your client. Ask one question, and wait for the response. Then, frame your next question based on the response you just got. Let your client lead you, rather than you hurling a handful of questions at him for him to sort out. Pauses and moments of silence are acceptable and can be very therapeutic. Consider the pause between his response and you developing your next question or statement as part of the process.

When in doubt of what to say next, just insert a pause. Sometimes a client will use those silent spaces to reveal something. When you are quiet and thinking about what to say or do next, you might suddenly hear your client continue on to the next step on his own. This is what you want to have happen with SomaCentric Dialoguing. You have succeeded in helping your client tune in with his body. Encourage him with words such as "And…," giving him permission to elaborate more. Tell him, "Yes…," acknowledging that you have heard him and that he can keep going. "Interesting" and "Tell me more" are additional phrases to use to continue the dialoguing.

Those silent times are powerful, sometimes just as powerful as asking the perfect question. Two other ways that silence or pauses can be therapeutic are with Pregnant Pauses and a concept I call "putting a client on pause."

Pregnant Pauses

Sometimes not saying anything is just as powerful as asking the perfect question. This is where Pregnant Pauses are used. Your client may answer your question with a Pregnant Pause at the end. For example, when you ask "How does this feel?" or "Is the pressure okay?" she might respond with "Fine…" and leave something unspoken. This is a Pregnant Pause. Sometimes Pregnant Pauses might sound as if she could continue with the word "but." When this happens, respond with "and…" It gives your client permission to add more or continue on with other information. It provides her with the opportunity to tell you something is done or enough.

The next time your client responds to a question of yours and seems to trail off and not finish or have a long silent pause at the end, dangling from her answer, encourage her to continue or add more information by saying "and…" or "yes…"

Putting clients on pause

Refer back to chapter 10, "Getting Started," where you learned the Permission technique. A key part of this technique is to allow your client the opportunity to have a quiet space to feel, to give himself permission to feel what is going on in his body. The technique of putting your client on pause is similar.

Sometimes your client will be caught up in his mind or brain, as he tells you the "story." As he does this, he does not allow himself to connect or be in touch with what his body wants him to be aware of. Another situation occurs when your client describes so articulately what he notices in his body that he rushes past any body-centered sensations that are also present. In both cases, your client does not allow himself to feel, does not give himself the time or space or permission to notice sensations. His words describe what is going on, but he does not experience what he describes. He avoids the situation. This avoidance may be conscious, or it may very well be the doing of his unconscious. "It's too scary to feel that, so I'm better off to just rush past any opportunity to feel."

This is where your skills as a therapist who knows how to listen to your own Indicator Compass or follow the compass readings come in. What you want to pay attention to is the question "Is my client physically aware, feeling the sensations that arise in his body, as he is describing what he is aware of?" If you answer, "Yes, he feels what is going on," then the session is proceeding in a good direction. If the answer is "No" or "Maybe he is not in touch with what is going on but is just talking about it," then it becomes your job to slow your client down and get him in tune with the sensations in his body.

You can very easily slow your client down by politely interjecting a comment: "I want to interrupt here a moment." Make a mental note of what he just said. You may need to refresh his memory later to start back into the dialoguing.

Inform your client that you would like him to pause a moment. The reason you are pausing him is to give him the opportunity to feel what is occurring in his body. Simply say, "I want to put you on pause for a moment." Then pause for a moment yourself before you proceed, to show what you want him to do. Continue with, "I want you just to pause a moment and allow yourself to feel what just happened in your body when you said _____." Fill in the blank with what he said when you felt your Indicator Compass clue you in that he had skipped over something.

He may not have been aware of what he just said that was important for him to sense. You may have to "rewind" what he said. Go back a little in the dialogue to just before your Indicator Compass went off. Repeat back to him, as close to verbatim as possible, what he said: "You just said _____." As you are repeating this information to him, pay attention to your sensor. Let your client know when it goes off, "Yup, right there. Yes, just be with that."

Depending upon his response, you can continue with the instructions of "I want you just to take a moment and feel that." If it is something that is significant and seems important for him to become fully aware of but he is trying to skirt around it, use the Permission technique with him at this time.

It is important to remember that a client needs space and time to get in touch with sensations, messages, and occurrences in his body. If he rushes past awarenesses, he misses pieces that could be very beneficial to his healing process. Putting your client on pause allows you to slow the session down and redirect and refocus him on what he has skipped over.

CLUES—NOT IN BODY SENSATIONS

Along with your Indicator Compass, there are other clues you need to be aware of to make sure your client remains in her body-centered awareness and does not disassociate. A client disconnects or disassociates from her body, or a part of it, as a response to something unpleasant, which is often triggered by trauma or the reexperiencing of a traumatic experience. The aim of SomaCentric Dialoguing is to help keep your client connected and in tune with her body. Therefore, it is important to know the clues or indications that she may not be in her body. Some of them are the client:

- has eyes open wide, perhaps is staring
- has drifted into another world
- uses the word *think*
- says, "My mind says..."
- turns to look at you, the therapist, for affirmation
- goes off on irrelevant tangents
- talks in an overly clear narrative, like reading from a script
- says, "That's scary to consider"

Eyes open

Quite often, a client will open his eyes or have kept them open as a means to reduce his awareness of his internal processes. This is not always true, however, for visual processors. A client who processes information visually may need to have his eyes open to help get in contact and sort what it is he is feeling within his body.

If a client has his eyes open and it seems as if he wanders, does not stay on track, or avoids something, use the techniques you learned in chapter 6, "Dialoguing," where dialoguing was discussed. If needed, pause the dialoguing to bring him back into his body sensations. Use techniques that focus on bringing your client's awareness into his body. Invite him to feel the weight of his body securely supported by the table (or chair) below him. Invite your client to take some deep breaths. Check in with him to make sure he is feeling safe and make sure you are still creating and holding a safe space. Invite him to bring his awareness back into his body, maybe in the area where he was previously or maybe in the area of your hand contact.

Once he is back in body-awareness, resume the dialoguing where you left off. It is okay if you are unsure of where you left off. It is acceptable to pick up the session by asking your client to describe what he is now currently aware of or to follow any comments he may be making as he gets back into his body-awareness.

Drifts into another world

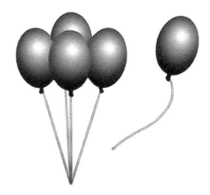

Picture yourself dialoguing with a client, and there is a long pause in the dialogue. Pauses are normal and acceptable and often therapeutic. However, this pause you are experiencing does not end. Your client's energy feels different and has shifted in some way. If you were to describe the situation, you might say that your client has spaced out or become disconnected or has drifted off somewhere. Drifting off is sometimes a protective mechanism to avoid feeling a past trauma. Sometimes it is an avoidance technique in which your client's unconscious prevents her from becoming aware of something in her body. Falling into a state of semi-sleep is another way with which a client drifts off and out of touch with her body.

Whether it is a protective mechanism and still beneficial, an avoidance technique, or just falling asleep, bring your client's awareness back into her body. The simplest way to do this is to call her by name, emphasizing her name at the beginning of a question or statement. If you want to know what she is aware of under your hand, which is on her arm, ask "Georgia, what are you aware of under my hand?"

If your client continues to drift off multiple times throughout the session, it could be an indication that it is a protective mechanism. She needs to get her conscious mind out of the way for benefits to be received during the session. Check in with your Indicator Compass to decide if this is a therapeutic state for her. If this happens and you are a bodyworker or manual therapist, just shift the focus of the session away from dialoguing to doing manual or energetic therapy and allow your client to be in the place to which she has drifted. If you are not a bodyworker, determine what is appropriate for your professional situation. You might allow your client to doze for the remainder of the allotted time, or you may choose to wake her up and give her the choice of continuing awake or ending the session.

Uses the word "think"

When your client uses the word *think*, it is a clear indicator that he is moving his awareness out of his body and into his head. As previously discussed, *think* is a word to be avoided because it requires the brain to engage and to analyze the situation or question being posed. The brain knows quite a bit, but in SomaCentric Dialoguing it is the body that needs the client's attention.

Avoidance or disconnecting from his body is evidenced by your client's making statements about what he thinks. When you hear this word, it is a clue to you that you need to help refocus him into his body sensations. Sometimes a client will briefly get caught off track, and, if you catch it early, it is very easy to help him redirect his focus back on his body.

Mind says

Another indication that your client is analyzing, rationalizing, or thinking is when she uses the phrase "Well, my mind says..." If you pay attention to your Indicator Compass when she says this, you will probably notice a change. The figurative compass needle will probably start to swing away from a clear "yes." When your client tells you, "My mind says...," it does not indicate that what she tells you is inaccurate; rather, it indicates that she is processing what she is aware of from a brain/mind-centeredness rather than a body-centeredness.

The phrase "Analysis creates paralysis" fits here rather well. Your client's mind knows quite a lot, but you want to keep her focus on her body-awareness. When this happens, especially if you feel the compass needle shift, ask her if her mind or her body is talking: "Was that your mind or your body just now telling us...?" Or "Who was that just now, your mind or your arm [body part being worked with]?" You may need to inquire a couple of times before your client, her mind, and her body get the message that you want to work only with her body at this time.

Sometimes the mind really has a lot to say, which is often the case. If this happens, I thank the mind for showing up and wanting to help out. I inform it that we really want to know what is happening with my client's body part, naming the specific part. If necessary, I allow it a moment to say whatever it wants and then step aside. If that is not enough, I send it to Hawaii (see chapter 11, "Meet the Twins") until we need it back.

Turns and looks at you

Similar to using the word *think*, your client may turn and look at you to receive confirmation about something he just did or said. This may be an indication that he is processing in his brain what is happening, rather than just allowing his body to communicate and experience. Your client may turn to look at you because he is unsure about what it is he is supposed to be doing. He might believe that you are looking for a particular answer or response, and so he looks at you for guidance or acknowledgment that he has said the right thing.

If your client looks for guidance or affirmation, inform him that there are no right or wrong answers. Let your client know that his best answers come straight from his own body, unedited and uncensored. Sometimes it is difficult for a first-timer to trust what he is getting. Sometimes he believes that he is making up the responses. Inform him that you want to hear the first thing that he is aware of, without his altering or filtering it.

Bring him back into his body and help him get back in tune with what his body wants him to be aware of. This is an appropriate time to give a couple of small indications that he is doing well. When he articulates what his body is communicating or what he is noticing, affirm that this is exactly what is most helpful for him.

Later, after the session, take the opportunity to educate him more about the validity of his first responses. If appropriate, tell him about how the session changed and got back on track once he started trusting his gut responses or instincts. If you have read the book *Blink*, let him know one or two things you learned from the work, such as about the art expert who could determine, the moment he saw a piece of art, whether or not it was a fake. And there was the tennis coach who knew the moment a ball was hit if it would go out of bounds, before it even hit the ground.

Goes off on an irrelevant tangent

Tangents can be important. Some of them are key and crucial to follow. However, sometimes your client may go off on a tangent that indicates that she is no longer in touch with her body-awarenesses. These are tangents that are irrelevant. Your Indicator Compass will help you determine this. Other ways to determine if your client has taken you on the start of a wild-goose chase is if the topic is totally unrelated to the previous dialogue. Of course, irrelevant tangents are sometimes a breather and can be therapeutic by creating a little space before your client goes back into the more difficult situation about which she is dialoguing.

If your client has gone off on a tangent and you are not sure about the therapeutic value, allow her to wander a little. Follow the dialogue for a minute or two. Keep track of where your client was when she went off on the tangent, because you may need to help her get back on track. When it becomes apparent that she is just talking around or avoiding something or needs to take a little break, allow her the space to do so. Then, gently ask her to come back to the place just before she began to talk about the unrelated tangent.

You may need to give her a couple of words or a sentence or two as a prompter. If you are unsure, you can rephrase what you heard her say. This is a good time to use Wiggle Words with your statements to get her back on track. Using Wiggle Words allows her to correct any inaccuracies of what you have said.

Appears to be reading from a script

Similar to going off on tangents, a client who is not in his body will often dialogue and describe what he is aware of as if he were reading a narrative or script. This script comes from his brain, not his body. It is a story; often it has been told time and again. Often it is what he tells family, friends, doctors, and talk therapists. You will sense the difference between your client's narrative script and his body's talking.

Here is the analogy that I like to use: you have a friend who just talks on and on and on. All you hear in your head is "Yadda yadda yadda yadda yadda" continually. You have heard the story before even if the words are slightly different. But one day this same friend tells you something that comes across in a very heartfelt way. Her words may be similar to those of her usual talks with you, but the intention and energy behind what she says are very different. In the first situation, your friend just spews words; she does not speak from body sensations. With the second situation, she comes from a deeper place within her body. The difference is very noticeable.

Quite often a client is unaware of the difference. He has his story, and he wants to be heard. You need to decide how much time you have and how important it is for you to listen to his story. More than likely, his story has been listened to before. The question yet to be answered is whether his body has been listened to. More than likely, his body has something it needs to communicate.

Be sure to honor your client's story before you proceed. Honoring his story may be a verbal acknowledgment, or it may be a nonverbal and energetic acknowledgment. Your job is to negotiate a way to move your client beyond the script he is telling you and get him in touch with what his body wants to reveal. This needs to be done tactfully, since sometimes a client really needs to have the opportunity just to narrate his script.

A diplomatic way is to inform him that you are there to help him get in touch with his body. You, the therapist, are interested in hearing what his body wants him to be aware of. From there, use the techniques you learned in chapter 10, "Getting Started," about beginning a session and bringing his attention into his body. You may need to use the 10 Things or the 1-2-3 techniques to help him get started.

"That's scary to consider"

The last clue I want to describe is this: when a client is disconnected from her body-awarenesses, she might say something like, "That's scary to consider." *Consider* is another word for *think*. The process of consideration requires her brain to analyze what is going on. Avoid asking, "What do you mean?" Asking her "What do you mean?" brings her more out of her body and more into her head. You want to turn her focus more to her body. If your client tells you that something is scary to consider or "I don't want to go there," it is a big bull's-eye sign saying here is the target. When this happens, continue to hold a safe space and give your client permission to feel what is happening in her body. Then, use any appropriate technique to help her listen to her body and determine what her body wants her to know.

RESTATING/REFRAMING STATEMENTS

An important and easy way for you, the therapist, to indicate to your client that you are paying attention and understanding what he is saying is by restating or reframing what he has expressed. The difference between restating and reframing is that, with restating, you are repeating as closely as possible what your client has said. With reframing, you are taking the key points or concepts about which your client has dialogued and rephrasing them into a synopsis of the dialoguing. It is also an important and helpful skill to develop in case the client gets off track. When you restate or reframe what a client has said, it is important to use Wiggle Words. You need to make sure you provide your client with the opportunity to correct you and change anything you might not have stated correctly.

Restate when you need to give your client a reminder about where he got off track. It is easier to restate what a client has said if you pay attention to what is happening in the session and in particular to what is said. It is helpful to remember the last sentence or two that has been spoken because restating will be easier if you remember what he has said as exactly as possible. This takes some practice, so do not be discouraged if you are not able to do it immediately. Wiggle Words allow you the opportunity to get something wrong: "Correct me if I'm wrong, but I believe you said…"

Reframing what has occurred in a session can be particularly helpful when a client has gone from one item to another and on to additional topics. Reframing is a good way to give your client a brief description of the progress or direction the session has taken. "It seems to me, and please change my words if you want, that after _____ happened, then you became aware of _____, which resulted in _____ happening." Reframing is a good way to affirm that you have been paying attention and witnessing the client's process.

Restating, reframing, or acknowledging is a form of witnessing. Many times a client may have done a lot of talk therapy about forgiveness connected with a traumatic experience. She may have done a lot of logical processing of a situation. Sometimes in the process, though, she may have not felt that someone witnessed her experience. When you restate and reframe, you witness her and her body's healing process. This occurs without any judgment and avoids analyzing what your client has said.

"SHOULD" VERSUS "NEXT TIME" OR "CAN"

In chapter 3, "Key Concepts," the concept of keeping a client in her body-awareness by having her employ the present tense was discussed. Similar to keeping the client's dialogue in the present tense, it can be therapeutic to ask the client to use particular words.

How many times have you said to yourself or someone else, "I should have done _____"? I hear this from clients on a regular basis. The use of the word *should* implies that he did something wrong because he chose the wrong action. Using *should* also does not move the client forward in action; it keeps him locked into the past. An alternative to the word *should* is the phrase *next time*. "Next time I will _____." This acknowledges that he could have done something different and that he is open to making a different choice in the future. Another alternative to *should* is *can*: "I can do _____." This helps your client reinforce that he is capable of doing something different in the future.

WHO/WHAT/WHEN/WHERE/HOW—CAREFUL WITH WHY

SomaCentric Dialoguing is all about helping your client get in touch with what is happening in her body. Help her do this by focusing her attention on what a part or parts of her body feels, looks like, and sounds like. In chapter 3, "Key Concepts," I used the analogy of painting a picture by starting with abstract images and filling in details as the session progresses. Sometimes you may get to a point where more information would be helpful. What can you do if the dialoguing does not naturally flow to fill in the details?

Have your client fill in the details easily with the use of who, what, when, where, and how (WWWWH) questions. Take, for instance, a situation in which your client has given you a couple of descriptions of a part of her body. There is more, but the next obvious question does not automatically come forth. Begin to ask her who, what, when, where, and how questions: "Who put it there?" "What was happening when you first became aware of it?" "When did you first notice it?" "Where in your body is it stored/held?" "How big [small, heavy, dark, etc.] is it?" Simply take the information your client has told you and expand upon it with WWWWH to facilitate further description and explore what is going on in her body.

As you ask these who, what, when, where, and how questions, be careful of "why." It is your turn to now ask me, "Why?" "Why" brings your client into his head and out of his body. Be careful of asking your client why something is a particular way. Avoid "Why is it red?" This asks him to analyze why the part of his body is red. The answer might be mundane and logical, such as because he is describing his heart, red refers to the blood that runs through it. But if he describes his heart as black and you ask, "Why is it black?" he may not have the answer. Black might be the first impression that came to him. Black is important information, but he needs to avoid analyzing it.

You want your client to stick with the first impression that came to him. For him to answer "why" implies that it may or may not be the correct answer. Remember: there are no right or wrong answers. To answer why questions allows him to rationalize what he is aware of and can often create defensiveness. If he goes on the defense, he may not feel safe. You want your client to feel safe.

Use who, what, when, where, and how questions to fill in the details of your client's awarenesses. Keep your client in his body by avoiding why questions. Avoid why questions to discourage analyzing or rationalizing his awarenesses and descriptions.

IS IT IMPORTANT?

Quite often, when we are busy and our children want our attention, we ask, "Is it important?" Sometimes, in therapy, it may not be clear if an aspect of the situation being explored needs to be filled in further or answered. Pay attention to your Indicator Compass to help you know if what has been said needs more attention and should not be overlooked or set aside. What has just been said could be key, or it could be a minor detail with little importance. If my Indicator Compass starts to make the compass needle wiggle, I ask, "Is it important to know?"

Quite often the dialoguing will be like this:

> *Therapist*: How long has it been with you? [This could be any question.]
>
> *Client*: A long time.
>
> *Therapist*: How long?
>
> *Client*: A very long time.

Therapist: A year, five years, ten years, thirty?

Client: I'm not sure, just a long time.

Therapist: Is it important to know how long it has been that way?

Client: Yeah.

Therapist: Okay.

> *Then proceed to give client some guidance on how to fill in the details about how to determine how long it has been there.*

Or

Client: I'm not sure, just a long time.

Therapist: Is it important to know how long it has been that way?

Client: No.

Therapist: Okay.

> *Continue on as normal.*

Is it important to know the story? Is it important to know what it is about? How long that feeling has been there?

This knowledge might help your client, or it might not. Your inquisitive nature may want to know more. Remember that it is not about *you* knowing all the details of the story. The therapist's job is to help the client determine what is important to be aware of for her healing. Be cautious here since figuring out the details of an aspect might keep the client in her head. Use your Indicator Compass to help you and your client determine how important it is to fill in particular details of the story.

ARE WE THERE YET?

Has it ever seemed as if you do not get anywhere, but you trust that progress is being made? Sometimes a client has to go through the struggles or revisit a situation before he can make his big "Aha!" There have been many sessions where 45 minutes have gone by, and it seemed that we just went around in circles or got off track on to tangents. Then, suddenly, my client came to an important awareness, realization, or understanding. Those few moments were all that were necessary to connect the dots and tie up the session.

- "Are we there yet?"
- "She'd better hurry up, or we'll be out of time."
- "What am I not doing right? We're not getting anywhere."

When these questions pop into your brain and you know that you have been doing your best, you need to trust. Trust your client's process. There have been many times when it seemed as if there was not enough time after the "Aha!" to bring the session to a nicely wrapped closure. That is okay. There is no rule that says that the session has to end on a high note, with all loose ends taken care of and tied with a pretty bow.

Let me tell you about Margie, a client who experiences bladder spasms. Quite often she has to use the bathroom in the middle of a session. At first, she was hesitant to do any dialoguing, lest she have to stop and interrupt the session. She thought it might ruin the session. I informed her that by no means did her getting up to use the bathroom impede the session. "We just press the pause button for the session and resume when you come back in." That sounded okay with her.

During her second session, she tried diligently to make it through the entire hour. She did not know how long she had been on the table. She did not know that I was looking at the clock, thinking, "She isn't close to resolving this and we're almost out of time." I trusted her body and her process that we were almost done. Then, she said she needed to use the bathroom. Her bladder was screaming to her when it reached the 50-minute mark. "That's fine. Thank you for taking care of yourself by saying something," I said.

When she came back, I gave her the option of extending her session by another half-hour at an additional cost or of taking the next five minutes to wrap up the session. "Let's finish up now; I got the most important part resolved." From my perspective, she had actually worked on many important parts to her situation. We wrapped up the session in the next five minutes. After she got off the table, I asked her for her comments. She was fine. She felt that the session was complete.

I informed her that, anything that was not tidily finished, her subconscious could keep working with to bring about resolution. I suggested that she honor any memories or emotions that might arise later during the next few hours or day. That sounded fine to her.

You will do fine if you trust your skills, speak with clarity and confidence, and trust your client's healing wisdom.

A LOVE STORY

Like any good love story, there are three characters involved, the two in love and the mutual friend. There are also emotional elements of love (duh—otherwise, it would not be a love story), hate, mistrust, and, quite often, jealousy. Also, there is a lot of communication or lack thereof. The love story that I will tell you about is one between Head and Heart. There are two mutual friends in this story—Client and Therapist. The premise of this story is that Client one day says to Therapist,

"Head knows and does everything; however, I think Heart wants more of this relationship." Therapist says, "Let's see what we can do."

Therapist: What part of you knows about this situation?

Client: Head knows all about it.

Therapist: Okay. And what part of your body knows about this situation?

Client: (*Pauses. Thinks. Pauses again.*)

Therapist: (*Waits patiently for a response.*)

Client: I think my heart. Yeah, that's it—my heart.

Therapist: Okay. Tell me more about what you notice about your heart.

Client: Well, I think it is lonely.

Therapist: Tell me more.

Client: (*Pause*) It is lonely and shriveled and shivering.

Therapist: How long has it been this way?

Client: (*Pause*) It seems like for ten years.

Therapist: Was that Head or Heart speaking just now?

> The words think *and* seem *can be words to clue you into the fact that the responses may not be body-centered, but may in fact be coming from the head. Pauses are clues that rationalizations, thinking, and second-guessing by the head may be going on.*

Client: Umm, that was Head.

Therapist: Hi, Head. Is there something you want to tell us about this situation?

Client/Head: Yeah! That silly Heart just doesn't get it. I keep telling Heart that being nice is not going to get it anywhere in this world.

Therapist: That's interesting. Heart, did you hear what Head just said?

Client/Heart: Yeah…but…

Therapist: But what?

Client/Heart: But no one listens to me, so I've just tried to make myself as small as possible.

Therapist: Well, you've got Client's attention now. What would you like Client to know?

Client: Client had better toughen up or else Client is going to have some real difficulties at work.

Therapist: Head, is that you again?

The Indicator Compass started wobbling to clue in that it might not be Heart speaking.

Client/Head: Yes.

Therapist: If it's okay with you, we'd like to talk with Heart for a little while. We'll then come back to you, as I know you have a lot of information.

Client/Head: Well, okay, but I'm going to be listening in to everything Heart has to say. It's my job to keep Heart out of trouble.

Therapist: Head, you're welcome to pay attention. Heart, are you still there?

Client/Heart: (*Softly*) Yes, I'm still here.

Therapist: What would you like Client to know? You've gotten Client's attention.

Client/Heart: Well, Client's work is tough enough as it is, and bringing home the problems just makes my job harder.

Therapist: What is your job, Heart?

Client/Heart: It's my job to hold compassion and empathy and sympathy and caring. But Client opens up my doors and lets all the emotions of the job in and out each and every day. That's really exhausting for me.

Therapist: Keep going.

Client/Head: I keep trying to tell Client not to work so many hours, but Client doesn't listen to me.

Therapist: Head, is that you again?

Again, the Indicator Compass clues Therapist in that Head has butted in. Also, there is a detectable change in tone of voice as each individual part speaks.

Client/Head: Yeah—okay, I'll be good and let Heart speak.

Therapist: Thank you, we'll get back to you. Heart, what happens when Client lets all those emotions in and out?

Client/Heart: Well, I get tired, and then I can't do my job of holding caring and compassion and empathy and sympathy.

Therapist: Then what happens?

Client/Heart: I start to run out of steam and stumble.

Therapist: And what happens to Client when you run out of steam and stumble?

Client/Heart: Client gets tired real easily, doesn't have time for family or friends, and is grouchy.

Therapist: Heart, what will happen if Client keeps going like this?

Client/Heart: Client is going to get really sick and won't be able to work.

Therapist: Heart, what would you like to tell Client?

Client/Heart: I need you to slow down, not work so many hours. I need you to limit your case load and not get so emotionally involved with your patients.

Therapist: Client, did you hear what Heart just said?

> *Even though Client is doing the dialoguing and speaking, asking her to confirm what she just heard from her body helps her to more fully get the message her body wants her to be aware of.*

Client: (*Sighs*) Yes, I did. I know I work too much.

Therapist: Heart, what else would you like Client to know?

Client/Heart: A vacation would be a really good idea—now, not in three years. We haven't had one in over ten years. Client only stops working when Client is sick, and that's not a vacation.

Therapist: Client, did you hear that?

Client: Yes. And Heart's right. I keep saying "Well maybe next year…"

Therapist: Heart, what will happen differently in Client's life if Client slows down, doesn't have too many cases, and goes on vacation?

Client/Heart: (*Cheerfully*) Client will have more energy and be healthier.

Therapist: Heart, with Client slowing down and having more energy and being healthier, then what can happen?

Client/Heart: Well, for beginners, with having more energy and more time, Client can exercise more, and Client will not be grouchy. And I will be able to hold a lot of caring and compassion in me to share with patients, family, and friends.

Therapist: Client, did you hear that?

Client: Yes.

Therapist: How would that feel, Client, to have more energy and be able to exercise more and have more caring and compassion for your family and friends?

Client: That would feel good.

Therapist: What would good feel like?

Client: Soft, full, warm. Mmmm. Real nice.

> *Therapist has just helped Heart inform Client and Head what the possible alternatives are—keep working and get sick and be grouchy, or slow down, have energy, and feel soft, full, and warm. It is very helpful to have the body part that knows about the situation, Heart in this case, show Client and the rest of the body what could possibly happen. A lot of resolution has occurred at this point, so even if the session ended here, Client would have gained a lot of benefit from the session.*

Therapist: Head, are you still there?

Client/Head: (*With attitude*) Of course! It's my job to keep everyone safe. I've been listening to every word.

Therapist: What would you like to say to Heart?

Client/Head: Well, first off, if Client doesn't keep a full case load, then the work doesn't get done. And Client gets lazy if Client isn't working.

Therapist: Describe lazy.

Client/Head: Lazy as in not productive, sits around, makes small talk, and just hangs out.

Therapist: Who does Client sit around and hang out with?

Client/Head: Well, no one when I'm in charge. But Client would be hanging around with the kids all the time if Heart had its way.

> *Some negotiations between involved parties clearly become needed when finger-pointing and blaming start showing up.*

Therapist: Head, what is the worst-case scenario that would happen if Client hung around with Client's kids?

Client/Head: Nothing would get done.

Therapist: Nothing? That's interesting. Do you mean to tell me, and please correct me if I'm wrong, that if Client slowed down a little, only took the basic case load, and hung around with Client's kids, nothing would get done?

Client/Head: (*Sheepishly*) Well, maybe not nothing. Just not as much as I'd like.

Therapist: Heart, please tell Head what you told us would happen if Client doesn't slow down.

Client/Heart: Head, Client is going to get really sick and not be able to work at all if Client doesn't slow down.

Therapist: Heart, do I understand you correctly that if Client doesn't work a little less that Client won't be able to work at all?

> *Restating and using Wiggle Words are important to help keep accuracy and clarity of the message.*

Client/Heart: You got it.

Therapist: Head, did you hear that?

Client/Head: Yes. But I really don't like the idea of Client's not keeping up.

Therapist: Head, would it be okay with you if Client tried it for a month? Just tried it for a month, until March 1, and then the three of you reevaluated the situation?

Client/Head: We could try it, but I'm not too sure how it will be.

Therapist: Heart, would that be okay with you?

Client/Heart: Absolutely!

Therapist: Client, would it be okay with you if, for a month, you only took the basic case load and hung around with your kids?

Client: It might take a couple weeks to discharge those extra cases, but then after that, I could try it for a month.

Therapist: Head and Heart, does that work with you?

Client/Head/Heart: (*In unison*) Yup!

> *At first glance, it may seem as if Therapist has offered a solution. Therapist has only reframed what Heart wants—for Client to slow down. Therapist has introduced some parameters, a trial period for a specific time period followed by a reevaluation. The key is that Therapist has made sure that these parameters are okay with all parties. If a party is not okay, help negotiate a resolution that is acceptable to all.*

Therapist: Client, is there anything you would like to say to Head or Heart?

Client: Head, thank you for doing such a good job watching over us. Heart, I'm sorry I haven't listened to you more.

Therapist: Head, is there anything else you would like to say at this time?

Client/Head: Just that I want them to know I'll be paying close attention.

Therapist: Heart, is there anything else you would like to say?

Client/Heart: Thank you for listening.

Giving each party—Client, Head, and Heart—an opportunity to say any last words and thank you's is a polite way to close and to put a nice bow on the session.

SURGERY PREP TECHNIQUE

As I have stressed throughout this book, the purpose of SomaCentric Dialoguing is to help your client get in touch with her body-centered awareness. Quite often, your client's body will have a difficult time healing because her body has had a scare or shock during surgery. One of the easiest ways to prevent a problem or surgical complication is to help your client ready herself for the surgery. I call this technique "Surgery Prep" because it is a wonderful way to help your client prepare her body for surgery.

Use this technique for any type of surgery or procedure. You can use it as preparation for tooth extractions or fillings, minor outpatient procedures, or something as complicated as hip replacement or brain surgery. It is particularly helpful to alleviate fear that stems from prior procedures or complications. There are no limits as to its use. Assign this technique as homework for a client before surgery.

If your body knows what is going to happen, then it knows what is normal and expected. Knowing what is normal and expected allows your body to relax and not have its guard up constantly. This provides more physical, emotional, and energetic reserves to be available should something out of the norm happen.

The concept is simple, and the technique is easy to use. Create a daily communication between the body and the mind. At least once a day, the mind needs to tell the body what will happen. The mind has a great wealth of information, and now is its time to share that information.

Your client needs to find out as much detail about what is going to happen in her procedure. Then, she needs to tell her body on a daily basis what will happen in the proper sequence of events and why. The client also needs to inform her body about the desired outcome. It is helpful to use other senses such as visualizing and feeling what will happen.

Providing the body with information ensures fewer surprises, so there is less against which it has to defend and protect itself. If it knows that something in particular will happen, then the body does not need to be protected from a surprise, and the body does not need to put protective mechanisms in place. If protective mechanisms are put in place, they might need to be negotiated with in the future, as described in chapter 11, "Meet the Twins."

To prepare

- The client explains to her body the procedure from start to finish.

- She is to use as much detail as possible because each detail is important and no detail is too mundane.

- She is to put the details in sequence as much as possible.

- She is to explain who is going to do each step, how it is going to be done, why it is going to be done, and what the desired outcome is.

For example,

1. Get up in the morning because you need to be at the hospital by 9 a.m.

2. Do not eat or drink anything because the doctors need your stomach empty so you don't throw up breakfast.

3. Get dressed because to go to the hospital naked would be cold and possibly embarrassing.

4. Go to the hospital/outpatient clinic. That is where the procedure will happen.

5. Check in so that the hospital staff know you are there.

6. Go to the surgery prep room so the staff can take care of you.

7. Get your vitals taken—blood pressure, temperature, pulse—so the nurses can tell the doctor that everything is fine to continue.

8. Talk to the nurse, doctor, anesthesiologist, etc.

9. Change into a dressing gown so you don't get your clothes messed up.

10. Lie on the presurgery bed waiting to be wheeled in. Hospitals don't like people walking around—the staff would rather push you.

11. Be wheeled in at the appointed time to a room that is white with bright lights. The lights are bright so things are able to be seen clearly.

12. Lots of people are there including the doctor and anesthesiologist. Everyone who is supposed to be there is there to help.

13. Be transferred from the bed to the operating table.

14. Have intravenous lines put in so the staff can administer the anesthesia and other necessary medications easily.

15. The nurse prepares the surgical site to prevent bacteria from creating problems.

16. The anesthesiologist tells you to start counting backward from ten to zero as he administers the anesthesia, so that you don't feel the procedure.

17. You become drowsy and fall asleep so time flies by and you don't feel anything unpleasant.

18. The medical team does its job well because each person is an expert and knows what she is doing.

> *The client describes in as much detail what will happen after the client's particular procedure and why it is happening.*

19. The staff transfers you to a regular bed and wheels you into the recovery room because you are all done and it's more comfortable in the recovery room.

20. You wake up nice and refreshed because the procedure went smoothly and the anesthesia was effective.

I know that it may seem trivial to include some of this information. However, when the body knows about something in advance, it can prepare; and when it is prepared, it can relax. After going through a narrative like the one above a couple of times, your client can eliminate some of the less important aspects. The most important parts are the details about what will happen during the actual procedure and why.

I used this technique myself when I had a minor outpatient procedure. Each day, for about a month prior to my surgery, I told my body what was going to happen, why it needed to happen, and what I wanted the outcome to be. I told my body what was happening on the morning of my surgery as I lay waiting in the pre-op room. I was wheeled into the surgery room, I was anesthetized, and my surgery was done. I had told my body that, after I was wheeled into the recovery room, I would sleep a little and then wake up nice and refreshed, relaxed, and pain-free.

After I was wheeled into the recovery room, I slept and dreamt. At one point, I heard a voice clearly say, "Julie, you can wake up now. It's time to wake up." So I started to wake up. The nurse saw me stirring and came over. "Oh, you're awake already. That's the quickest I've ever seen someone come out of recovery."

I was slightly confused. "Didn't you tell me I could wake up now?"

Looking around the room to see if anyone else was there, the nurse said, "No, I didn't say anything. I was over at the nurses' station when you started waking up."

Who told me I could wake up? I do not know for certain. However, I do know that I woke up refreshed and relaxed, just as I had told my body previously.

JUST BECAUSE TECHNIQUE

Assigning "homework" helps motivate clients to do things, such as exercising. As a bodyworker, I have assigned many women the homework of foregoing high-heel shoes because of the stress that they can put on the back. Clients love the excuse of "My therapist told me that I have to go buy new shoes because I can't wear my heels." One day, while SomaCentric Dialoguing with a client, a gremlin tried to tell her that it was not acceptable for her just to sit and watch the birds. Her gremlin wanted her to be doing something productive at all times. Inspired by that session, I designed a homework assignment in which my client would give herself permission, despite her gremlin's objections, to do "nothing."

I see clients continually stressed over how they have to be on top of the housework, keeping everything neat and tidy, spic and span and spotless. I see clients who are so driven and such diligent, hard workers that they rarely take time to stop and smell the roses. I hear from their bodies about the toll that it takes. Their bodies need them to take a break. However, their gremlin or brain will not go for it. From these situations, I developed "Just Because." Just Because is a self-care tool. It is about learning how to do something or nothing for no reason whatsoever. Just Because is about doing something or nothing without having to justify it.

If during a SomaCentric Dialoguing session it has been revealed that part of my client's body wants her to slow down or not work so hard, I assign Just Because as homework. Just Because is about giving my client permission to do nothing if that is what she feels like doing. It is about giving her permission to buy herself some flowers for no reason at all. When my client has a gremlin that is causing difficulties and makes her justify everything she does, sometimes a little practice is needed to help her feel comfortable doing something for no reason at all—doing it just because.

I encourage you to get creative with how the Just Because technique can be used by your client. Have her brainstorm about all the things her body wants her to enjoy but that her brain or gremlins will not allow her to unless she has a good reason or excuse to do it. When someone has to use the excuse of "My husband wants to go on vacation, so I guess we'll finally take one for the first time in ten years," then this is a good indication to take a just-because mini-vacation. Help your client get away from the justification of doing something because of someone else. Encourage her to do something for herself.

Societal beliefs are such that a person should not enjoy something unless she has a good reason; otherwise, she is being selfish. This is not accurate. Taking care of oneself goes beyond just providing food, clothing, and shelter. Taking care of oneself includes finding a healthy balance between work and play, between responsibilities and just kicking back. Life is meant to be enjoyed; when the body starts sending messages that it is time to slow down, listen to those messages. Have your client do some Just Becauses as a wonderful way to help her reeducate her body and brain that life will not end but will be more enjoyable and less stressful.

Just Becauses can be large and complex like taking a vacation for no reason at all, or they can be small and simple like taking a walk. I encourage my client to do one Just Because each day. For maximum benefit, I ask her to do something different each day. This helps her learn to expand her sphere of comfort. If she prefers to do the same thing each day, that is acceptable as well. A Just Because can be a one-time event such as calling a friend, or it can be an ongoing activity such as taking a class in watercolor painting. Eventually, your client will realize that she can do one or more of these things each day and still be productive in her daily life.

Here are some client indications for using Just Because:

- has a difficult time justifying doing something for herself
- needs a reason to do something
- needs permission just to enjoy life
- believes that if she does not have an excuse to do something, she should not do it
- needs to learn how to do things without having a reason
- does not know how to enjoy the simple things in life

What are some of the types of things to do just because? How about the following?

- buy flowers
- take a walk
- read a book
- watch the birds

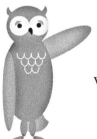

JUST BECAUSE EXERCISE

What other types of Just Becauses can you think of?

13 *Creating a Session*

SomaCentric Dialoguing is easy—that is, if you understand the concepts and principles that I have described as well as the purpose and flow of the individual techniques. However, it can be confusing, disconcerting, or even scary at times. Questions therapists often ask me when they start learning SomaCentric Dialoguing are "Am I doing it 'right'?" "What next?" "Can I hurt my client?" The most pressing question most therapists have is "How do I start?" This chapter will help you put the pieces together from start to finish.

FRAMING THE SESSION
First, you need to know your client's intention for the session. I call this framing the session or setting the intention. Why is my client coming for help? Why is she here? What is her chief complaint? During the client interview, I can get a good idea of the answers to these questions. With a returning client, I like to find out how she felt after her last session, as well as what she wants help with in the current session. I use the information that I have gathered at the beginning to help guide my client through the session. At the end of the session, I help her connect the dots and realize the value of the session.

During the time of this first interaction, I pay attention to what communication language the client speaks. Is he a Red, Blue, Green, or Brown or a strong combination person? I also pay attention to what his processing style is. Is he more visual, kinesthetic, or audial? His words tell me how he perceives, thinks, communicates, and expresses himself. I make a mental note about the languages he speaks. I begin immediately to use my client's same language as I converse with him.

After I complete my intake with a new client or a brief check-in with a returning client, I say something like, "All that being said [acknowledging the conversation and intake information from client history], if there is one thing I can help you with today, what might that be?" This is the most important question to be answered because the structure of the session is determined by what the client wants help with.

Sometimes a client says she wants help with a physical problem, and the session reveals an emotional component that holds back her healing. Sometimes it is the other way around. Sometimes there is a physical problem or stress that is causing an emotional problem. Sometimes the "one thing" is different from her initial chief complaint as listed on her client-history form. And until the end of the session, it may not be apparent how the client's "one thing" actually is related to the chief complaint.

Sometimes a client asks if he can have "two things." I allow him to do this. Often, unbeknownst to him, the two things are related. Having him identify what he most wants help with allows the situation(s) to come into his conscious awareness more completely. Once he has answered the question of "one thing," I generally have a couple of ideas regarding how to start the session, so he then climbs onto my table. If you are a therapist who is not doing table work, this is where your client would get comfortable in the chair or on the couch.

SESSION OPENING

I start all my sessions with my client on the table, lying comfortably on her back. I then gently cradle her head in my hands and begin the session by saying the following:

> *I'd like you to begin this healing session*
> *by taking some nice, deep breaths, in and out, bringing in the breath, fully and completely,*
> *allowing it to flow to every cell of your being.*

> *And as you let the breath out,*
> *allow your body to let go,*
> *letting go of anything not needed at this time.*

> *Bring in the breath,*
> *allowing it to nurture you, guide you, and heal you;*
> *and as you let the breath out,*
> *allow your body to just melt, unwind, let go.*

> *If at any time*
> *anything is uncomfortable, just let me know,*
> *as this is a safe space for you on your healing journey.*

I do this opening recitation for a variety of reasons. First, it allows my client and me to tune in energetically with each other. It allows us a constructive opportunity to focus our attention on being centered and breathing. As a bodyworker, I am also beginning to tune in to what is going on physically in my client's body. Second, the words that I say have a specific purpose. If I were to say this opening recitation to you, you would probably feel your body beginning to relax. You will notice, however, that there is no use of the word *relax*. Instead, I have asked you to allow your body to let go of anything that is not needed, to allow your body to melt and to unwind. I do not use the word *relax* for all the reasons I talked about "No-No Words" in chapter 8, "Word Choice."

In this opening invitation, I have my client focus his attention on his breath, bringing it into his body and into his cells. Not everyone is able to do this easily. I want my client to begin to tune in with his body as soon as possible. To focus his attention immediately on his breath brings him out of his head and the thoughts he walked in with into his body and his body sensations.

I have him bring in the breath and instruct him that it can nurture him, guide him, and heal him. This helps him know on a subconscious level that healing can begin simply with his breath.

Repetition is important as well. Repeating words and phrases helps deepen the message that I want the client to receive. I tell her a couple of times to breathe in and out. I want her to do this consciously a couple of times so that she deepens her state of relaxation. You will notice that I also use the phrase "let go" or "letting go" three times. Repetition is necessary to help your client get the message that she has permission to let her body release anything that it does not need.

I begin to empower her when I tell the client that she should let me know, at any time, if she feels uncomfortable. Letting her know that this is a safe space helps her to know on a subconscious level that she can allow her defenses to lessen.

There is an addition that I sometimes include with this opening:

> *If at any time any thoughts, images, memories, emotions, or sensations arise, feel free to explore them, either verbally out loud or quietly to yourself.*

When I use this statement, I insert it before the last phrase, "If at any time anything is uncomfortable, just let me know, as this is a safe space for you on your healing journey." This optional addition invites my client to begin the dialoguing on his own. It gives him permission to pay attention to what is happening in his body. It tells him it is okay, even helpful, for him to express, describe, and explore what he is aware of, out loud.

One day a client arrived late, and I did not have any free time scheduled immediately after her, so we needed to have a shorter session. She talked a lot as she got on the table, so I thought I would just skip this session opening. I put my hands under her head to tune in with her body. As I searched for the opportunity to begin dialoguing with her, I started doing some bodywork. She immediately said, "Aren't you going to hypnotize me?"

"Hypnotize" was the best word she could think of to indicate that my opening words helped her to relax and slow down. It had helped her to settle during each session I had done it with her. Her question "Aren't you going to hypnotize me?" expressed how important it was for her to begin her session with the opening I had always used.

A couple of years ago, I moved across the country; I closed one practice and opened another. Before I moved, I asked a couple of my clients who had been with me for about three years if they got benefit from hearing this opening invitation each time they had a session, sometimes weekly. They all said that they enjoyed it, as it really helped them to be calm, be centered, and relax. They all looked forward to this "recitation" or "invitation" as a structured way to help them get into a relaxed state. My clients' responses confirmed for me how important it is to set the tone of the session as a safe space, to connect with each other, and to begin to bring my client into her body.

BEGINNING THE DIALOGUING

In chapter 10, "Getting Started," I discussed how to get dialoguing started with your client. Here again is "How to Get Started," an abbreviated version:

1. With your hands on your client, ask her to bring her awareness to where your hands are.

2. Ask her to get a good sense of that area.

3. Ask her to get a good sense of what is or is not going on in that area.

4. Ask her to notice where her attention is being drawn.

5. Say, "Let me know when you have a good sense."

6. When you get acknowledgment that she has a good sense of the area, ask her, "What are you aware of?"

7. From there, just follow the trail she gives you.

If she gets stuck, offer the client suggestions with lots of Wiggle Words:

"Get a good sense of what it looks like, what it sounds like, what it feels like."

"If it were to have a color, what would it be?"

"If it were to have a shape, what would it be?" *or*

- texture to touch

- size

- smell

- temperature

- sound

- name

You can ask, "If there is one place in your body that knows all about the situation, where would it be?" Or you can have the client answer the question by using various techniques that were previously discussed, such as Mini Me, 1-2-3, and 10 Things, to bring his attention to the area of his body that wants to communicate. These are ways to begin having your client tune in with his body. These techniques help him to begin putting words to his sensations and articulating his awarenesses. Be creative, and trust your client's healing wisdom.

If your client has difficulty tuning in with or articulating what she is aware of in her body, consider using the Permission technique. This technique gives her the opportunity just to notice and be aware of what is happening, without having to put words to it. Sometimes a client has never felt she had permission to notice or feel what her body wants her to know. Sometimes the Permission technique needs to be used for only a minute or two to get things started. Sometimes it may become a large part of a session. Follow your client's body, and pay attention to your Indicator Compass.

Keep in mind

Help your client explore an area(s) that wants attention by using open-ended questions and nonleading, nonjudgmental questions. Communicate in and use words that are in your client's processing/communication language(s) – Red, Blue, Brown, Green, audial, visual, kinesthetic. Where appropriate, have her build on all three processing languages (audial, visual, and kinesthetic) to help deepen her healing at a subconscious level. Keep in mind throughout the session to use Wiggle Words and be aware of your word choice—*discomfort* rather than *pain*, or *sense* rather than *feel*. When you want to rephrase or restate something your client has said, reflect back what your client stated, using her own words, or as close to them as possible. When you notice the reason for a difficulty, make appropriate adjustments to your dialoguing.

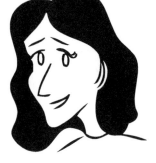

If you experience difficulties go over this checklist:

- Are you speaking the client's language?

- Is the client in her head/mind/thinking, or is she in her body?

- Are you asking appropriate questions? (nonleading, nonjudgmental, open-ended)

- Does the client speak using "I" rather than "you"?

- Is the client having difficulty because she does not know how, does not know what is expected?

- Is resistance or a protective mechanism coming up?

- Do you need to "give the client permission" just to experience or be aware of what she is feeling/sensing?

As needed and as appropriate, use the other techniques from various chapters. You might wind up using a couple of different techniques. You might use one technique to help your client locate and identify where the difficulty is in her body. For this purpose, you might use the Mini Me, 1-2-3, 10 Things, or Permission techniques. Then, you might use another technique to bring about resolution. Other techniques to use are Bodyguard Job Reassignment, Guardian Angel, and Safe Space Conversation.

Surgery Prep and Just Because are two unique techniques. These are ones that I use with a client for self-care and infrequently during a session. They are described in chapter 12, "Gems and Nuances."

WRAPPING IT UP

When time is almost up, begin to close the session both energetically and verbally. As I mentioned in the previous chapter, "Gems and Nuances," Margie had to get off the table to use the bathroom before we were done with her session. When she got up, we had only a little bit of time left, but it seemed that more work could be done. By energetically shifting the focus and intention from exploring to concluding, her body was informed that it was almost time to end. It is similar to knowing when you have been over at a friend's house long enough. Her energetic interaction with you starts to change.

You can also verbally begin to wrap up the session by letting your client know that he has done a lot today, that there are only so many (use a precise number) minutes left in the session, and that this would be a good time to start drawing things to a conclusion or to an end. A way I like to do this is to offer his body the following opportunity: "In the next three minutes, which is all the time in the world for the subconscious, allow your body to finish anything it needs to." It is amazing what happens.

Then, when there is closure to the session, I put the bow on it with my closing recitation, similar to the opening:

> *I'd like you to begin closing this healing session*
> *by taking some nice, conscious, deep breaths in and out,*
> *bringing in the breath fully and completely into your body.*
> *And as you let the breath out*
> *allow your body to fully let go,*
> *letting go of anything that's been released.*
>
> *Bring in the breath,*
> *allowing it to continue to nurture you, guide you, and heal you.*
> *And as you let the breath out,*
> *allow your body to fully let go of anything that's not needed anymore.*
>
> *Begin to become conscious and aware of the sound of my voice,*
> *and the touch of my hands,*
> *bringing yourself back fully refreshed and revitalized,*
> *knowing that you can return to this state of peace, relaxation, and healing*
> *at any time.*
>
> *There you are.*
> *Thank you.*
> *Take your time getting up.*
> *I'm going to go wash my hands, and I'll be back in a minute.*
> *Take your time.*

In the second-to-last stanza, I begin to increase the volume of my voice. I have previously spoken in a soft tone but now begin to get a little louder and more articulate. I also begin to contact my client with my hands in a firmer manner. With my voice, I put emphasis on the words *can* and *any*. I do this to emphasize that the client is able, he is capable, even if he does not know it, to return to this state of peace, relaxation, and healing. And he is able and capable of doing it at any given time. It does not have to be only there in my office on my table. He can do it at home or at work or while traveling. Clients have told me over and over that they will hear my voice or imagine me saying this to them when they are stressed or injured, and it helps to bring them back in to a peaceful and healing space.

I have also told my client that the session is over. I have told her what is expected of her—she is to take her time getting up. I have told her she has permission to take her time, that she does not have to jump right up off the table. I prefer that she does not jump up. I tell her to take her time because I want her to allow herself really to tune in and be aware of what is happening (or not happening) in her body in a fully conscious state. With this last stanza, I have also told her what I am going to do. She now knows that I am going to leave and then come back.

I leave the room to wash my hands. I use this as an excuse to give her alone time. With no one around, she can begin to process more easily what has occurred. She knows what is expected. She does not have to react immediately to my watching her. Nor does she have to be concerned that I might immediately ask her something. I find that a client stays more fully with the sensations that she is aware of in her body by giving her this time.

END OF SESSION

When I come back in the room, I first check in with my client. I say something like, "Thoughts, comments, questions?" Other things I might ask are "What do you notice?" or "What is different?" With great expectation, I sometimes ask, "So…" I speak this way because I want to ask a very broad, open-ended question. I want to know what thoughts my client has about the session. She might have a comment to make, and I want to give her permission to speak it. I want to let her know that I will answer questions. I use the phrase "Thoughts, comments, questions?"—instead of asking "How are you?" or "How do you feel?"—because I want to avoid the standard trite, nonbody-centered answers of "Fine" or "Good." This phrase allows and gives my client permission to:

- tell me how she feels (good or bad)
- ask any questions that might have come up during or immediately after her session
- make any comments that are milling around in her head
- tell me anything else that she wants

The phrase "Thoughts, comments, questions?" also gets you a lot more feedback from the client than if you were just to ask, "So how are you feeling?" She might want to know what you felt. She might want to know more about this type of therapy. She might want to know if SomaCentric Dialoguing [fill in the type of therapy you do] is good for [*fill in the blank*] because her best friend has x, y, or z. She might want to refer a friend, and so on. It is a great way also to help build your practice.

If my client does not have much to say about the session, I then ask her, "What do you notice that is different?" This question helps her to start tuning in with something that may be different from when we started the session. My goal is to get her to pay attention and realize as many differences and changes that have occurred as she can.

When she tells me something like "I feel softer" or "looser," I then use that piece of information to fill in the blank of the next question: "Now that you are feeling looser/you have softened, what can happen differently in your life?" This question makes her think about how she can have beneficial changes in her life:

> *Now that _____ has happened/you are feeling _____, what can happen differently in your life?*

Sometimes I follow up the client's response with another, similar question, "And when [her answer from previous question] happens, then what can happen?" This allows her to realize even more how her life can be different. When I ask my client this question, I get her to stop and think about what can occur, what can be improved and be better. When she answers this question, really wonderful changes start to happen in her mind and in her body and can occur more easily in her life. I encourage you to use these questions. They help ground the work and the changes that have transpired in your client's body. They can make a huge difference in the long-term results of a session. It also helps the client to get a good sense of the value of the work.

When a client has indicated the results were what he wanted to achieve, sometimes I ask playfully, "Mission accomplished?" Even though this is a closed-ended question, it can be used to help my client say, "Yeah! That was great!"

Here are other examples of how to use the question "Now that something has changed, what can happen differently in your life?" Use your client's processing language to reinforce how she can get better in touch with her body-centered awarenesses.

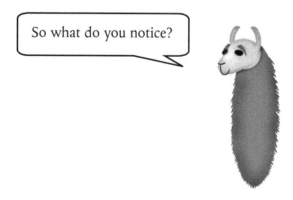

Therapist: "Now that your heart feels more open and light, what can happen differently in your life?"

Client: "I can feel more love and let more love in."

Therapist: "And feeling more love and letting more love in, what can happen differently in your life?"

Client: "I can have a better relationship with my boyfriend. Yeah, he'd really like that…"

Or

Therapist: "Now that you hear what is causing your stomachaches, what can happen differently in your life?"

Client: "I can listen better to my body and realize when I can let go of needing complete control."

As I discussed in the beginning of this book, where it is appropriate, help your client connect the outcome of the session to the initial intention. When connecting the dots for her, if and only if it is necessary, reflect back to her any awarenesses she experienced. Help your client link her initial intention with the session's occurrences and outcome. As always, be sure to use your client's own words without interpreting or projecting any judgment. And use Wiggle Words when you do this.

Was the chief complaint different from the "one thing" the client specified she wanted help with? Did your client make the connection? Did she have this awareness during or at the end of the session? If yes, then remind her of the connection. Use as many of her own words as you can. If no, that she did not make the connection herself in the session, you can advise her in a manner such as, "Over the next little while, maybe between now and the time you leave, or later this evening, I invite you to explore the connection between [satisfying self with food] and [being physically accosted]."

Or you might propose how the chief complaint might be connected to the outcome of the session, using lots of Wiggle Words: "I'd like to toss this idea out to you. If it works/resonates great; if it doesn't, that's fine. [Giving permission.] You initially came in for [state chief complaint] and when I asked you if there was 'one thing I could help you with,' you mentioned [fill in the blank]." From here, continue to ask her if she is aware of a correlation or connection. If she is, then ask her, "Mission accomplished?" or "Did we achieve what you hoped?"

If the client still does not have an awareness of the connection, then use lots of Wiggle Words as you continue further: "Does this resonate?" Continue cautiously with your perception of the connection. Be careful not to make judgments or analyze the situation. Use the client's own words and phrases without leading her or changing the meaning of her words. Do not read too much into the situation or project your own beliefs, issues, and judgments.

Remember:

- Do not jump to making the connection for the client.

- The client may need to work at making the connection.

- It is acceptable to leave the client pondering.

- the Gurdjieff quote about the difference between knowledge and understanding. (see chapter 3, "Key Concepts.")

- Let the client make the connection.

CASE SESSION

Here is a session that I did with Karen during her second appointment. She told me that the one thing I could help her with was to identify and understand why she felt "off." We put her on the table; I cradled my hands under her head and started to tune in with her. I said my opening invitation: "I'd like you to take some nice, deep breaths…" We start the dialoguing immediately with my first question of "What is going on?" I specifically refer to her intention.

Julie (me): What is going on?

> *I refer to her intention.*

Karen: Something is "off." I can't put my finger on it.

Julie: How many weeks has this been going on?

Karen: Three.

Julie: What is going on in your life?

Karen: I just moved my office. I am learning new work, which, I'm finding, is all that I want to do. It feels like this new work is my calling.

> *We explored this a little bit, then moved on.*

Julie: What else is going on in your life?

Karen: I'm missing my grandparents.

> *Karen told me that, within the last two years, she had lost both of her grandmothers and that she really missed them.*

Julie: Where in your body do you feel that sense of missing your grandmothers?

Karen: In my heart.

Julie: What does your heart feel?

Karen: Sadness.

Julie: How big is that sadness?

Karen: Grand Canyon size.

> *Without prompting or inquiry, Karen continued.*

Karen: Head doesn't want me calling Grandpa.

Julie: How do you feel when you do call Grandpa?

Karen: Glad. I'm glad when I do.

Julie: How big is that gladness?

Karen: Grand Canyon size.
> *We then spent some time with Head and Heart, determining what each knew and what each wanted to have happen or not.*

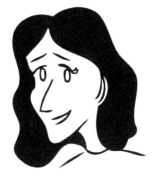

Let your client connect the dots.

Karen: I know that I need to listen to Heart.

Julie: How do you feel when you listen to Heart?

Karen: More grounded, happier.

Julie: How do you feel when you listen to Head?

Karen: "Off," missing something.

> *We spent time negotiating with Head and Heart about what needed to happen so that Karen could follow what Heart wanted to tell her.*

Karen: I miss talking with Grandma. I used to talk with her on the phone frequently.

> *We then began a Safe Space Conversation (see chapter 10, "Getting Started") with Grandma, so Karen could tell Grandma that she missed talking with her and all the wonderful things that were happening in her life.*

Julie: Do you want to talk with her in person or on the phone?

Karen: On the phone.

Julie: Describe to me where you are.

> *Karen told me that she was in her house, in the living room sitting on the sofa with her phone. This is where she often sat when she would call Grandma. Karen described the time of day and what she was wearing. This is done to help her place herself in the situation as completely as possible. She talked to Grandma, quietly to herself. I told her to let me know if she had any questions or needed any help. Periodically I checked in with her by asking, "How are you doing?" Karen told me, "We're still talking." Or she would say, "We're done now. We've hung up."*

Julie: How does Heart feel?

> *I inquire about Heart to tie the Safe Space Conversation back in to the previous dialogue about Heart's feeling sad because Karen missed being able to talk with Grandma.*

Karen: Grand Canyon feels filled in a little; I'll take that. (*Karen smiles.*)

> *Smiles or eyes lighting up are indications that the body has achieved a goal.*

Julie: Heart, anything else you want Karen or Head to be aware of?

Karen: No, I'm good.

Julie: Head, anything else you want Karen or Heart to be aware of?

Karen: Nope.

Julie: Karen, how do you feel when you think about calling Grandpa?

Karen: Good. (*Karen smiles.*)

Julie: Here's a thought that just came to me; feel free to use if you want or change it in any way [lots of Wiggle Words so Karen could claim this for herself]. What if, when you call Grandpa, Grandma listens in?

Karen: That would be okay. (*Karen smiles again.*)

> *After these feelings have begun to settle in, we close the session, "I'd like you to begin closing this healing session by taking..."*

After Karen got off the table, she reported that she felt wonderful, like something had lifted. What could happen differently in her life? She said that she could enjoy her talks and visits with Grandpa more and still be connected to Grandma by envisioning Grandma's calling her.

A couple of weeks later, when I saw Karen next, she told me that she still felt as wonderful as she had immediately after her session.

14 *Getting Unstuck*

I have answered the question of "How do I start?" Now, I will gaze with soft eyes into my crystal ball and see your next question: "What do I do if I get stuck?" This is an important question and I am glad you asked. Any self-respecting "how-to" book needs to cover this and other similar, trouble-shooting questions. Here are some scenarios where you might consider yourself stuck.

"WHAT IF MY CLIENT DOES NOT KNOW HOW TO DIALOGUE OR DOES NOT WANT TO?"

Please refer to chapter 6, "Dialoguing"; this question is covered in detail there.

"WHAT IF I DO NOT KNOW WHAT TO SAY OR ASK NEXT?"

If you do not know what to say, just wait. To wait and to use a pause are very acceptable. Pausing is appropriate even when you do know what question to ask next. Trust that your client will say something or that the next question will arise naturally. If you still do not know what to ask, check in with yourself. Are you breathing? Your brain has a difficult time thinking and paying attention if you do not breathe freely. When you tense up, you might hold your breath. Your brain has difficulty getting oxygen when your breath is restricted, and that makes it difficult to think. So, make sure to breathe.

Make sure that you hold a safe space. Are you at ease, physically and mentally? If not, adjust your posture or the room so that you can hold a safe space and be relaxed. Your client may subconsciously pick up on your discomfort and try to protect herself by not dialoguing.

Do you hurry or rush your client? If so, just take a deep breath. Make sure you are grounded, are holding a safe space, and allow yourself to slow down. Follow your client's pace. If you rush your client or seem to be in a hurry, her subconscious will notice. She might interpret your rushing as "She's not able to help us" or "She's too busy with other things." If time is a concern, then politely address this situation with your client. You can easily say, "We have ten minutes left in this session, so I want to give you the opportunity to bring things to a place of closure."

Do you not know what to say or ask next because you are not focused on your client, but have let your mind wander? If so, refocus your attention fully on your client. Drifting will and does happen, especially when you first learn how to do SomaCentric Dialoguing. Mentally acknowledge to yourself what happened and use it as a reminder that you need to be attentive always of what is happening with your client.

"WHAT DO I DO WHEN MY CLIENT GETS CONFUSED?"

First, clarify the source of the confusion. Is the client confused because he does not know what to do? If so, refer to chapter 6, "Dialoguing." Is he confused because he has a difficult time focusing? Or is he disconnecting from his body? Make sure that you help focus him in body-centered awareness and not in a thinking-and-analyzing mode. Pay attention to any signs of protection and resistance, as described in chapter 11, "Meet the Twins."

Is your client confused because she has a difficult time being aware of what is happening in her body? To assist her optimally, make sure to use her primary processing language. If your client does not use an obvious audial, visual, or kinesthetic language, she might be a sensing processor. You will need to use broader words if she is a sensor, as discussed earlier in chapter 5, "Frustrated Aardvarks."

Is your client confused because you asked him the next question before he has finished responding to the previous one? Do you anticipate what you think should happen next? (The answer should be obvious.) Avoid jumping the gun. With SomaCentric Dialoguing, strive for being one step behind rather than two steps ahead of your client. He is the lead, so allow him to show you where he goes next.

Remember that the session is about the client, not what you think it should look like or be about. A helpful way to avoid jumping the gun and confusing your client is to allow a moment of silence between his answer and your next question. How long that moment lasts is up to you. Pause after he has answered your question. This allows his answer to sink deeper into his subconscious awareness. This helps deepen the effectiveness of the session. In this moment of silence, your client may add something that might change your next question. Follow his lead.

"I DO NOT KNOW WHAT TO ASK NEXT—I'M EITHER AT A DEAD END OR GOING IN CIRCLES."

If you are stuck in this position, it might be that your client has tried to lead you off the path or on a wild-goose chase. A wild-goose chase is often an indication that Resistance is present and does not want your client to become aware of something. Be diplomatic when dealing with that twin, Resistance. It might be Resistance that has led you down a dead-end trail. Or it might be that your client needed briefly to explore that particular trail. This is fine. Now, it is your job simply to backtrack to the place where she wandered off the path.

Does it seem like the client takes you in circles? This could also be Resistance poking its head into the session. Check it out. It could be that you did not pay attention to your Indicator Compass when the needle started to drift into the going-off-track zone. When the session goes in circles and you are speaking her language, simply pause and backtrack. Rewind the tape to a place close to where you went astray, and pick up from there.

Sometimes I say to a client, "It seems as if we're not getting anywhere. I'd like to propose, if it's okay with you [lots of Wiggle Words], that we back up a little to the place where you said…" I then name the place from where I would like her to continue. Usually, a client has noticed the circles and is happy to have some guidance about how to progress. If we are really stuck in a pickle jar, I might say, with ample Wiggle Words, "Okay, if it's all right with you, let's try this…" and I use a different technique. Otherwise, we work with a topic previously mentioned by the client, which shifts the direction of the session.

"I GOT DISTRACTED AND DON'T KNOW WHAT'S HAPPENING. WHAT SHOULD I DO?"

Occasionally, something like this happens. Maybe there was a noise outside your treatment room that caught your attention just as your client said something. Maybe your client began to mumble his response, and you could not understand it. It is possible that your mental shopping list diverted your attention away from your client. If this happens, acknowledge to yourself what happened and refocus on your client. If you are not clear about what your client last said because it was inaudible or unclear, simply ask him to repeat himself: "I'm sorry, what was that?" Other times I repeat back what I think he said, using lots of Wiggle Words, "Correct me if I'm wrong, I believe you said…"

If you have gotten thoroughly distracted and do not know what is happening or it seems as if something is happening quietly but your client is not revealing what is occurring, simply ask him "What are you aware of?" and continue from there.

"WE HAVE MORE TIME AVAILABLE, BUT NOTHING IS COMING UP. WHAT DO I DO?"

If an awareness and some level of resolution have occurred, then that might be all there is to be done for the day. Sometimes a client comes in wanting help with a multifaceted situation. Only one aspect of it may need to be addressed for complete resolution. It is okay not to complete it in a single session. Her body may indicate that it needs simply to process what just occurred and nothing more. Check in with your Indicator Compass, trust your client's healing wisdom, and do not force an agenda upon her.

"I'M NOT SURE ABOUT MY INDICATOR COMPASS."

It is essential to be able to follow your Indicator Compass. If you have difficulty, go back to chapter 3, "Key Concepts"; read over and explore the different ways therapists sense their indicator. Then, practice with some friends or other therapists in a situation where it does not matter professionally. It can also help to receive sessions or mentoring where the focus is paying attention to your indicator. The most common reasons for a therapist's having difficulty with his Indicator Compass are that he lacks clarity and confidence about his perception of yes and no. A tremendous boost comes from working to gain clarity in using your Indicator Compass.

"SOMETIMES I GET PANICKY AND BEGIN TO WONDER IF I SHOULD BE DOING THIS. WHAT THEN?"

Understand that being unsure is a very common reaction, especially when first learning SomaCentric Dialoguing. Feeling panicky is a common response to having a lack of confidence. As you gain more confidence with the techniques and learn how to utilize your client's languages, you will have less doubt and will not tend to feel panicky. A mentor can help you gain more confidence by talking with you about the session and how to improve your techniques.

As long as you keep your client grounded and focused on body-centered awareness, your sessions should flow well. Remember not to analyze or judge anything your client has said. You are there to help your client become more aware of what happens in her body, not to interpret what does or does not occur.

If you start to get panicky, remember to breathe and stay grounded. If your client is becoming agitated and uncomfortable, have her breathe and bring her awareness into her body. If she feels out of control, have her open her eyes, breathe, and come back into the room. She may have completed all that her subconscious needed for this time. Remember that a successful session does not mean it has to be wrapped up tidily with a nice bow. Regardless of how tidy and smooth a session appears, the goal of SomaCentric Dialoguing is to help your client become aware of what is happening in her body.

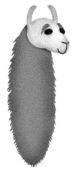

- Trust
- Wait—allow for pauses
- Listen to your "yes/no" Indicator Compass—what bearing is the compass reading: wandering/BS/ on track?

"WHAT DO I TELL MY CLIENT WHEN SHE ASKS HOW SOMACENTRIC DIALOGUING IS DIFFERENT FROM PSYCHOTHERAPY?"

In SomaCentric Dialoguing, the therapist learns to speak the client's language and helps him to be in touch with what is happening within his own body. The therapist does not interpret the client's situation in SomaCentric Dialoguing. SomaCentric Dialoguing focuses on the message that the client's body wants to reveal. He is the one who "connects the dots" of awarenesses revealed and derives his own meanings from the session. Psychotherapists often interpret the meaning of something that has been said; SomaCentric Dialoguing therapists do not. Psychotherapy is usually not body-centered, whereas SomaCentric Dialoguing is totally focused on the body.

15 *Techniques Review*

This chapter lists and reviews the structure of a session and the different techniques that you have learned throughout this book. At the end of this chapter, there is a brief review of the Success Signals communication styles and AVK processing styles. While all the material in this chapter will sound familiar, it has been abbreviated; I have omitted the descriptions and explanations of these techniques, so that it is easier for you to put the book beside you and refer to it throughout your session. Feel free to change the scripts of these techniques, as needed. (I have given you what works for me.) Alter the phrases to suit your professional style and the communication and processing styles of your clients.

SESSION STRUCTURE

Here are the different components of a session:

- Session flow
- Which twin: Protection or Resistance?
- Framing the session
- Opening recitation
- Closing recitation
- End of session: Client check-in

SESSION TECHNIQUES

Here are the techniques that are reviewed in this chapter:

- How to get started
- Mini Me
- 1-2-3
- 10 Things
- Permission
- Bodyguard Job Reassignment
- Guardian Angel
- Safe Space Conversation
- Surgery Prep
- Just Because

Things to remember:
- Are you breathing?
- Are you relaxed? Mentally? Physically?
- Are you grounded?
- Are you holding a safe space?
- Are you watching for projecting your own stuff?

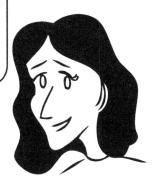

SELF-CARE AND HOMEWORK TECHNIQUES

These techniques can be used as homework or self-care for your client to work with on her own. They are easy to learn, especially after having experienced them during a session.

- Mini Me
- Safe Space Conversation
- Surgery Prep
- Just Because

SOMACENTRIC DIALOGUING SESSION FLOW

1. Do your client intake/history

2. Begin observing/listening/becoming aware of client's language:

   a. Success Signals—Red, Blue, Green, Brown

   b. AVK—audial, visual, kinesthetic, or sensor

3. Set intention for session:

   Ask, "If there is one thing I could help you with today, what would that be?"

4. Begin session:

   "I'd like you to begin this healing session by taking some nice, conscious, deep breaths."

5. Use various techniques to bring client's attention to area of body that wants to communicate:

   a. Mini Me

   b. 1-2-3

   c. 10 Things

   When appropriate, you can also use:

   d. Safe Space Conversation

6. Explore area(s) that wants attention using:

   a. open-ended questions

   b. nonleading, nonjudgmental questions

   c. words in client's processing/communication language(s): Red, Blue, Brown, Green, audial, visual, kinesthetic, sensor

7. Troubleshoot if you are having difficulties:

   a. Are you speaking the client's language?

   b. Is the client in his head/mind/thinking mode, or is he in body-centered awareness?

   c. Are you asking appropriate questions? (nonleading, nonjudgmental, open-ended)

   d. Does the client speak using "I" rather than "you"?

   e. Is the client speaking in present tense rather than past tense?

    f.   Is the client having difficulty because she does not know how, does not know what is expected?

    g.   Is resistance or a protective mechanism present?

    h.   Do you need to "give the client permission" just to experience or be aware of what she is feeling/sensing?

8.   Things to keep in mind throughout the session:

    a.   Use Wiggle Words

    b.   Reflect back what client stated, using her own words

    c.   Be aware of your word choice (for example, *discomfort* rather than *pain*, or *sense* rather than *feel*)

9.   When session time is almost finished:

    a.   begin to close session—energetically, verbally

    b.   check if you need to offer the client the opportunity to wrap up:

        "In the next three minutes, all the time in the world, allow your body to finish anything it needs to."

10.   Close session:

    Say, "I'd like you to begin closing this session by taking some nice, conscious, deep breaths."

11.   Check in with your client:

    a.   "Thoughts, comments, or questions?"

    b.   "What do you notice that is different?"

    c.   "Now that _____ has happened/you are feeling _____, what can happen differently in your life?"

    d.   Where appropriate, connect the outcome of the session to the intention set by the client at the beginning of the session.

    e.   If necessary—and *only* if necessary—reflect back to your client any awarenesses that arose during the session. Be sure to use the client's own words without interpreting, projecting, or judging.

Which twin: Protection or Resistance?

1.   Bring your client's awareness into her body.

    If there is difficulty doing this, refer to chapter 6, "Dialoguing," and the technique "How to Get Started" discussed in chapter 10, "Getting Started."

2. Give your client permission to:

- feel

- be there

   If necessary do the Permission technique with her, as described in chapter 10, "Getting Started."

3. Protection: Identify which category Protection falls into:

- current and helpful

- learned

- learned and helpful in past

- learned and helpful currently

- irrelevant

   If Protection is not currently helpful or beneficial and is no longer necessary, then continue helping your client identify it. It is now considered Resistance or a gremlin.

4. As described earlier, work with Resistance or a gremlin:

- identify it

- identify its purpose

- identify the message Resistance or the gremlin has

5. Have your client determine if Resistance is still needed. Have your client determine if any of it is worth keeping. Should she keep some of it or get rid of it all?

6. What does your client want to do with it? As described previously in this chapter, ask your client what she wants to do with Resistance. Below are some ways to help your client decide:

- Say, "Let me know if you need any help or would like a suggestion."

- Offer a variety of things other clients have done in the past. Use Wiggle Words when offering suggestions so that your client is empowered to make the situation her own.

- Does she want to give Resistance an eviction notice?

- Does she want to negotiate with Resistance?

- Does she want to offer Resistance a job reassignment: from being a bodyguard (24/7/365 on duty) to being a night watchman?

FRAMING THE SESSION

Have your client identify his intention for the session, to help provide a common focus for him and you. Based upon this intention, use the techniques that you, the therapist, have available to help your client achieve his goals. At the end of the session, help the client connect the outcome with his stated intention, to help him articulate how the session was valuable to him.

1. Setting the intention at the start of the session:

    - "Why are you here?"

    - "What is your chief complaint?"

    - "If there is one thing I can help you with today, regardless of the technique used, what might that be?"

    - "All that being said [acknowledging conversation and information from client history], if there is one thing I can help you with today, what might that be?"

        Sometimes the "one thing" is different from the client's chief complaint, but it is often related to the chief complaint or what initially brought the client in. However, this may not be apparent until the end of the session.

2. Revisiting the intention at the end of session:

    - "Thoughts, comments, questions?"

    - "Mission accomplished?"

    - Connect the dots

    - Tie in initial intention/goal with occurrences of session, and with the outcome

    If the chief complaint is different from the "one thing" and there is a connection, did your client have this awareness during her session?

    - If yes, she made the connection, then remind her of the connection, using as many of her own words as you can.

    - If no, she did not make the connection during the session, say, for example, "Over the next little while, maybe between now and the time you leave or later this evening, I invite you to explore the connection between satisfying self with food [intention for the session] and being physically accosted [resulting awareness from session]."

    - Using lots of Wiggle Words, you could also propose how the chief complaint might be connected to the outcome of the session, for example, by saying, "I'd like to toss this idea out to you. If it works/

resonates great; if it doesn't, that's fine. [Giving permission.] You initially came in for [state chief complaint], and when I asked you if there was 'one thing I could help you with,' you mentioned [fill in the blank]."

From here, continue to ask the client if she is aware of a correlation or connection. If she is, then ask her, "Mission accomplished?" or "So, did you get your money's worth?" or "Did we achieve what you were hoping for?"

If she still does not have an awareness of the connection, then use lots of Wiggle Words as you tell her your perception of the situation. Say, "Does this resonate...?" Continue cautiously with your perception of the connection, being careful of making judgments or analyzing the situation. Use your client's own words and phrases without leading her or changing the meaning of her words.

When doing this:

- avoid reading too much into the situation or projecting your own beliefs, issues, and judgments

- do not jump to making the connection for the client

- accept that the client may need to work at making the connection

- know that it is acceptable to leave the client pondering

- remember the Gurdjieff quote about the difference between knowledge and understanding

- let the client make the connection

OPENING RECITATION

See "Wrapping it up" in chapter 13, "Creating a session" for more information. Below is the way I begin my sessions:

> *I'd like you to begin this healing session*
> *by taking some nice, deep breaths in and out,*
> *bringing in the breath, fully and completely,*
> *allowing it to flow to every cell of your being.*

> *And as you let the breath out,*
> *allow your body to let go,*
> *letting go of anything not needed at this time.*

> *Bring in the breath,*
> *allowing it to nurture you, guide you, and heal you;*
> *and as you let the breath out,*
> *allow your body to just melt, unwind, let go.*

If at any time
anything is uncomfortable, just let me know,
as this is a safe space for you on your healing journey.

Below is an optional addition that invites dialoguing:

If at any time any thoughts, images, colors, or sensations arise, feel free to explore them,
either verbally out loud or quietly to yourself.

CLOSING RECITATION

See "Wrapping it up" in chapter 13 "Creating a Session" for more information.
To begin closing the session I say the following:

I'd like you to begin closing this healing session by taking some nice, conscious, deep
breaths in and out,
bringing in the breath fully and completely into your body.
And as you let the breath out, allow your body to fully let go,
letting go of anything that has been released.

Bring in the breath,
allowing it to continue to nurture you, guide you, and heal you.
And as you let the breath out,
allow your body to fully let go of anything that's not needed anymore.

Begin to become conscious and aware of the sound of my voice,
and the touch of my hands, bringing yourself back fully refreshed and revitalized,
knowing you can return to this state of peace, relaxation, and healing
at any time.

There you are.
Thank you.
Take your time getting up.
I'm going to go wash my hands, and I'll be back in a minute.
Take your time.

END OF SESSION: CLIENT CHECK-IN

Instead of asking "So, how are you feeling?" ask "Thoughts, comments, questions?" and go from there. This allows and gives permission for the client to

- tell you how she is feeling (good or bad)

- ask any questions that might have come up during or after the session

- make any comments that are milling around in her head

- tell you anything else that she wants

This question also gets a lot more feedback from the client than just asking, "So, how are you feeling?" She might want to know what you have felt, want to know more about this type of therapy, want to know if CST is good for [fill in the blank] because her best friend has [fill in the blank]. She might want to refer a friend, etc.

Another question to ask is "Now that something has changed, what can happen differently in your life?" This allows the client to realize how her life can be different. By asking your client this question, she has to stop and think about what can occur. What can be improved?

HOW TO GET STARTED

(See chapter 10, "Getting Started," for a complete description of this technique.)

1. With your hands[1] on your client, ask her to bring her awareness to where your hands are.

2. Ask her to get a good sense of that area.

3. Ask her to get a good sense of what is or is not going on in that area.

4. Ask her to notice where her attention is being drawn.

5. Say, "Let me know when you have a good sense."

6. When you get acknowledgment that she has a good sense of the area, ask her, "What are you aware of?"

7. From there, just follow the trail she gives you.

If she gets stuck, offer her suggestions with lots of Wiggle Words:

"Get a good sense of what it looks like, what it sounds like, what it feels like."

"If it were to have a color, what would it be?"

"If it were to have a shape, what would it be?" *or*

- texture to touch
- size
- smell
- temperature
- sound
- name

---

1   See chapter 10, "Getting Started," about modifying this for a non-hands-on session.

MINI ME TECHNIQUE

The Mini Me technique is a great way to start a dialoguing session. It is described fully in chapter 10, "Getting Started." If the concept of becoming aware of his body is new to your client, this helpful technique will introduce him to the concept of tuning in to his body. Use this technique when a client has a difficult time finding the area of his body that is trying to get his attention.

Below is what I say to my clients when using the Mini Me technique:

I want you to imagine reducing yourself to a mini-size.

Maybe you will use a machine similar to the one in the movie *Honey, I Shrunk the Kids*.

Or maybe you will use a special pill.

Or you simply may see or feel yourself getting smaller and smaller until you are a Mini Me.

Pause

Let me know when you are mini in size.

Pause

Once you are very small, I want you to find a way to get into your body.

Perhaps crawl in through your ear.

Melt and be absorbed into your skin.

Walk into your mouth and slide down…

Or you might just imagine yourself automatically shrinking into the center of your body.

Whatever works for you, use it to get inside yourself.

Pause

When you are inside yourself, let me know.

Pause

Now I want you to explore inside yourself.

Walk around.

Float around.

Feel where you are naturally drawn.

Pause

Find a place in your body that needs attention.

Allow your Mini Me to go to the place in your body that is wanting attention.

There may be a few places to which you are drawn.

If so, find the area that draws you most strongly.

Pause

If you need a flashlight to light your way, realize you have one in your hand already.

If you need a map to follow, it's in your pocket.

If you need a sign to show you, look up; it is right there.

Pause

Give your Mini Me permission to go wherever your body wants attention.

Pause

When you get to the area trying to get your attention, let me know.

Client indicates she is there.

Okay...

Now get a good sense of what is around you.

Pause

Where are you?

What are you aware of?

Tell me more...

Continue from this point of awareness having the client describe that area of her body. Use dialoguing to have her become aware of the message or reason that area of her body wants attention.

1-2-3 TECHNIQUE

See chapter 10, "Getting Started," for a full explanation of this technique. Use the 1-2-3 technique when your client has difficulty trusting what she is aware of or has a difficult time finding a starting place. The flash-pan-thought concept is used with this technique. Use the first thing that comes into your client's awareness as this is often significant. Remember that there are no right or wrong answers. The purpose of this technique is to help your client trust her body's responses and to establish an entry point for a dialoguing session.

Here are simple instructions to give your client:

I want you to close your eyes and just start noticing your body in general.

Take some deep breaths in and out.

As you breathe, notice your entire body as a whole, inside and out.

I'm going to count to three.

On three, you are going to tell me the first thing that pops up in your mind,

the first thing that comes into your awareness.

I want you just to go with it.

Allow the first thought to enter your mind without analyzing, censoring, or filtering it.

So, on three…

One,

Brief pause; then in a little firmer tone

Two,

Brief pause; then in an even firmer tone with authority

Three!

Pay attention to your Indicator Compass so you can help your client track if she is censoring her first response, should she try consciously or subconsciously not to acknowledge her first response.

What did you notice?

Tell me more.

Through dialoguing, help her explore what she noticed. Make sure to validate the client's experience by acknowledging that trusting the process might have been difficult. Using lots of Wiggle Words, help her connect the dots between her intention for the session and whatever her body wanted her to be aware.

10 THINGS TECHNIQUE

Use the 10 Things technique, as described in chapter 10, "Getting Started," when your client has a difficult time describing what he senses. Ask your client to describe ten things about the area that he wants to explore. This quick-and-easy way to start a SomaCentric Dialoguing session can be used when you are not sure how to help your client begin dialoguing. Additionally, use this technique if your client is having a difficult time determining the message his body wants to communicate. Working with this technique can be done in a short period of time, in only 5 to 15 minutes.

1.   These descriptions should be one or two words to keep his awareness in that area of his body and to prevent him from shifting into his head.

2.   Inform your client that you will keep count of how many descriptions he gives you.

3.   When appropriate, repeat back in the same order what he has said and let him know how many descriptions he has given you.

4.   As he proceeds, repeat back one word of the description that he has just said.

5.   As you keep track of how many things he has mentioned, tell him how many he has told you, as well as how many more he has to go.

6.   When he gets stuck, repeat back in the order given a number of his descriptions.

7.   Encourage him and help him stay focused in his body if he seems to be getting distracted or into his head.

8.   When he gets to his tenth thing, repeat the tenth one and then pause.

9.   Next, instruct him to give you one more. Instruct him to give you an eleventh. This is the most important description because, quite often, this is one he may have been trying to avoid telling you.

10.   This eleventh description is the one that you will have him explore in the session.

11.   From here, help your client explore what his body wants him to be aware of regarding the body part and any messages it may have for him.

PERMISSION TECHNIQUE

Use the Permission technique, as described fully in chapter 10, "Getting Started," when a client gets stuck, such as having a difficult time putting words to an awareness or is hesitant to articulate what she is aware of.

1.   Hold a safe space.

2.   Give your client permission to feel what she is aware of.

3.   Say, "Get a good sense of that area of your body."

4.   Pause…pause…pause.

   Pause between statements. Allow the client the opportunity to do what you have asked—to get a sense of her body. Pay attention to your Indicator Compass.

5.   Say, "Just give yourself permission to be with it."

Now it is time to give her, perhaps for the first time, permission to tune in with herself.

6.   Say, "Just be with it."

You are giving your client permission to be with it. Her being with it is more important than anything else at this point of the session.

7.   Rest with a long pause. Pay attention to what is going on with her.

8.   Say, "Give yourself permission."

9.   Say, "Give yourself permission to be with *that.*"

Repeating instructions clearly and simply keeps her on track.

10.   Say, "Get a good sense of it."

Even though you are repeating yourself, by just changing a few words, you can help her go deeper into her awareness.

11.   Say, "Yup. Just be there."

12.   Say, "Stay with it."

Repeat these or similar lines. These lines can be said in any order. When your client gets a good sense of "it" and she has given herself permission to be with it fully, feel it, see it, touch it, etc., then you can move on to having her explore the message that part of her wants to communicate.

BODYGUARD JOB REASSIGNMENT TECHNIQUE

As explained more fully in chapter 11, "Meet the Twins," the bodyguard is a protection mechanism that is on call 24/7/365. When trying to reduce this level of protection, it is helpful to suggest a job reassignment to that of night watchman.

Here is an example of the SomaCentric dialogue conversation between my client and myself:

Therapist (me): So you've identified a part of you that makes you edgy, jumpy, and on alert all the time. You have told me that you don't need this anymore and would like to get rid of it. Am I correct?

Client: Yes, that's right, but I don't know if I'm ready to let all of it go yet. It feels as if I need to keep some of it around.

Therapist: Okay. So, instead of having it around all the time, what if you gave it a job reassignment?

Client: Okay…

Therapist: For example, and you are welcome to use or change any of this, instead of having a bodyguard protecting you 24/7/365, walking around hovering over you all the time, what if you gave that bodyguard a job reassignment to a night watchman? He could have a chair and sit at a desk with lots of monitors to watch and make sure you are safe. He'd have a telephone to call for back-up. And he could have a radio if he needed to alert you about anything. And, if necessary, there could even be a big panic button he could press if he needs to get your immediate attention. But most of the time he could just sit there and kick back and eat donuts. How does that sound?

Client: That sounds good. I'd actually like him to _____.

   Encourage client to make any changes to fit her purposes and needs. Or if she has a different idea completely, use it.

Therapist: Okay, what I'd like you to do now is get a good sense of that part of you that has been your bodyguard. Let me know what you are aware of.

Client: Yup.

Therapist: Okay, what is your bodyguard's name?

Client: Bob.

Therapist: Okay, please say "Hi" to Bob, and let him know the situation. He's been working very hard, working 24/7/365 for _____ [specify amount of time]. He's been doing a really good job. [I only say this if I know he has been doing a good job based on what my client has told me.] And he's been making you feel _____ [however Resistance has made the client feel—tired, sick, unhappy, etc.]. Let him know that he doesn't have to work so hard anymore because the situation has changed and he is going to get a new and easier job. Let him know that he can now be a night watchman. Starting now.

Client: (*Either quietly to herself or out loud tells Bob all this information and then acknowledges when this has happened.*)

Therapist: Okay. How are you doing, _____ [client's name]?

Client: (*Responds accordingly.*)

Therapist: How is Bob?

Client: (*Responds accordingly.*)

Therapist: Anything else you two need or want to tell each other?

Client: (*Responds accordingly.*)

Therapist: (*Wraps up the dialoguing section.*)

Sometimes Bob the Bodyguard may not want to accept his reassignment for fear that he will not be able to act fast enough or get my client's attention. Some negotiations need to be done when my client wants to reassign the bodyguard, but there is reluctance on the bodyguard's behalf. One of the most effective ways to achieve this resolution is to let the bodyguard know that he can sit in front of a panel of television monitors that constantly watch my client. There is also a big, red panic button that he, as the night watchman, can press if he needs to get her attention quickly.

Sometimes additional communication tools are necessary to include, such as a special phone line or agreed-upon words or phrases to assure clear communication. Negotiating may require a couple of agreed-upon indicators for different levels of danger. A general warning may require a whisper in your client's ear: "Be careful." When the situation gets a little more dangerous., there might be a strong statement: "Keep your wits about you." Extreme situations might dictate that there be a shouting of "Danger! Stop!" Depending upon your client, the line of communication may need to be felt kinesthetically. This results in your client's experiencing a particular sensation in a benign manner, such as tingling in the left pinky finger or feeling as if someone were tapping on her shoulder.

GUARDIAN ANGEL TECHNIQUE

As described in chapter 8, "Word Choice," the Guardian Angel technique should be used when your client is in a position of vulnerability. Your client's guardian angel assists by providing information or intervention. This Guardian Angel technique can also be used when there is fear or your client is scared. When an aspect of your client, such as his inner child, needs to know something, use this technique to have the guardian angel provide him with information.

1. You begin by having your client identify a situation where he has expressed he does not feel safe (interpret this broadly).

2. Have your client get a good awareness of the situation.

3. Have him, if he is willing, describe the situation to you out loud. Having him tell you helps to deepen his awareness and keeps him from drifting off.

4. Have him describe to you how he is feeling, what emotions are connected to the situation.

5. Have him find out (from his body part, his little child, inner child) what he needs to feel safe, protected, and secure.

Quite often he will need someone to hold him (real or imagined, living or passed on), tell the offender something, or make the offender go away. Sometimes he needs someone to reassure him that he is loved, cared for, bright and intelligent, smart, wanted, etc.

6. Have him invite that person or being to be there with him.

    Sometimes this person is his adult self, who has learned a lot about life and has wonderful words of wisdom and the benefit of hindsight.

7. Invite the person to give your client any information or message that would be helpful for the given situation.

8. Have your client make sure that the part of him that is being spoken with and comforted really understands the message that he is being given.

    This is similar to the Permission technique. Sometimes your client will know what is being said to him, but it takes some time to sink in and absorb what is being communicated so that his body understands it.

SAFE SPACE CONVERSATION TECHNIQUE

As described more fully in chapter 10, "Getting Started," the Safe Space Conversation technique is helpful to use when a client wants to have a conversation with someone about a past event or future situation, but she is reticent or not able to speak directly with that person. During this conversation, your client can:

- tell someone how she feels/felt

- ask/inquire into why someone did/did not do something

- talk with someone about a potentially unpleasant future encounter/ event/conversation/meeting

- let someone know something

- have a conversation with someone who is deceased, not around for whatever reason, or incommunicado

- speak with someone she does not want to see in person, but needs to talk with

Here are the steps for this technique:

1. Find out with whom your client wants to talk and the general subject matter.

    Both the subject and conversation may change or shift as the session progresses. This is normal and acceptable.

2. Have your client visualize a safe space that:

    - is real or imagined

    - she knows, has been to, or knows of

    - she can picture or put herself there

3. Say, "Tell me when you are there."

4. Say, "Describe your safe space to me."

    This helps her fully to embody and place herself there.

5. Have the client get a really good sense of her environment and describe it.

    - (If outside) What season is it?

    - Is it sunny?

    - What is the temperature?

    - Is it breezy?

    - (If inside) Which room in the house is she in?

    - What furniture is there?

    - Are there windows?

    - What is she wearing?

    - Where is she sitting?

6. Ask, "Is there anyone you want there with you for support?"

    Inform the client that this support person may be real, alive, passed on, imaginary, a guide, parent, friend, or guardian angel. Be careful that you know her beliefs regarding guides and angels, etc.

    If the client indicates that she does not want a support person, tell her she can always ask for assistance to come in at any time.

7. Say, "Invite [name of person with whom she will converse] to come in and have a seat."

8. Have your client describe the features of this person:

    - hair and eye color

    - clothing

    - where he is seated

    By having your client describe the person with whom she will be talking, you help her get a full sense of the person.

9. Explain how the conversation will happen, using talking-stick rules:

    "You will go first. You get to say and or tell him whatever you want or to ask any questions.

    "While you are speaking, he will quietly be listening with open ears and full attention. He won't say or respond until you are done. Then it is his turn to speak, respond, and reply while you are quietly listening with open ears.

    "When he is done, you will get a chance to respond, answering any questions of his, replying to anything he has said. You may tell him additional things if you choose.

    "You will go back and forth until you are done.

    "So, go ahead. Tell him what you would like to know; ask what you would like to ask, while he patiently listens with open ears."

    If the client is speaking quietly, in her head, say, "Let me know when you are done."

    "Now it's his turn. What would he like to say?"

    "Let me know when he is done."

    Go back and forth until done.

    "Anything else you would like to say?"

    When your client is finished, say, "Thank him for coming and speaking with you and show him the way out."

    "So…thoughts, comments, questions?"

SURGERY PREP TECHNIQUE

This technique, described fully in chapter 12, "Gems and Nuances," is one of the easiest ways to prevent a problem or surgical complication and helps your client ready herself for the surgery. Assign it to her as daily homework prior to surgery. Use this technique for any type of surgery or procedure. It is particularly helpful to alleviate fear that stems from prior procedures or complications. There are no limits as to its use.

To prepare

- The client explains to her body the procedure from start to finish.

- She is to use as much detail as possible because each detail is important and no detail is too mundane.

- She is to put the details in sequence as much as possible.

- She is to explain who is going to do each step, how it is going to be done, why it is going to be done, and what the desired outcome is.

JUST BECAUSE TECHNIQUE

This is a homework assignment, described fully in chapter 12, "Gems and Nuances," that enables my client to give herself permission, despite her gremlin's objections, to do "nothing." It is about learning how to do something or nothing for no reason whatsoever. Just Because is about doing something or nothing without having to justify it. Have her brainstorm about all the things her body wants her to enjoy but that her brain or gremlins will not allow her to unless she has a good reason or excuse to do it. Just Becauses can be large and complex like taking a vacation for no reason at all, or they can be small and simple like taking a walk. I encourage my client to do one Just Because each day. For maximum benefit, I ask her to do something different each day. This helps her learn to expand her sphere of comfort. If she prefers to do the same thing each day, that is acceptable as well. A Just Because can be a one-time event such as calling a friend, or it can be an ongoing activity such as taking a class in watercolor painting. Eventually, your client will realize that she can do one or more of these things each day and still be productive in her daily life.

Here are some client indications for using Just Because:

- has a difficult time justifying doing something for herself

- needs a reason to do something

- needs permission just to enjoy life

- believes that if she does not have an excuse to do something, she should not do it

- needs to learn how to do things without having a reason

- does not know how to enjoy the simple things in life

What are some of the types of things to do just because? How about the following?

- buy flowers

- take a walk

- read a book

- watch the birds

SUCCESS SIGNALS COLOR STYLES REVIEW

This information is presented fully in chapter 4, "Talking Colors."

Remember that each person is a blend of these communication styles. One is not better than another. People have a tendency to have one color be dominant. If your client is a different primary color than you are, find that color within you so that you can communicate successfully.

Table 1. Success Signals communication styles

Red	Blue
Intuitive more than analytical	Intuitive more than analytical
Nonlinear	Asks for input
Spontaneous	Empathizes and shares testimonials
Enthusiastic	Considers how others will be helped
"No rules"	"Hugger"
Class clown	
Green	**Brown**
Analytical more than intuitive	Analytical more than intuitive
Logical	Logical
Asks for details	Gets to the point
Linear thinkers	Wants specifics
"Tell me more"	"Just do it!"

AVK PROCESSING LANGUAGE REVIEW

This information is presented fully in chapter 5, "Frustrated Aardvarks."

Audial

People who are audial or aural receive information through the sense of hearing. Phrases an audial client will use in her mannerisms of speech include the following:

- I hear...
- It sounds like...
- What comes to me...
- I sense...

Questions you can ask an audial client include the following:

- If it could speak, what would it say?

- What does it want to tell you?
- What does it sound like?
- Is it loud?
- Does it sound soft?
- Does it sound angry/sad/silly? (some emotion)

Visual

Visual processors are those who receive information through images. Phrases a visual client will use in his manner of speech include the following:

- I see…
- It looks like…
- When I look at it, I…
- It's red…
- It's big… (this can also be kinesthetic)

Questions you can ask a visual client include the following:

- What does it look like?
- If you were to look at it, what would you see?
- What color is it?
- What size is it?
- Tell me what you see.

Kinesthetic

People who are kinesthetic are those who feel. Phrases a kinesthetic client will use in her mannerisms of speech include the following:

- I feel…
- It feels like…
- If I touch it…
- It's hot…
- It's hard/rough/smooth… (can also indicate visual processor)

Questions you can ask a kinesthetic client include the following:

- What does it feel like?

- If you were to feel/touch it/pick it up/hold it, what would it feel like?
- What is its texture?
- What is its temperature?
- How big is it? What is its size?

Sensor

People who are sensors speak a little of one language, a smidgen of another, with a strong flavor of vagueness. Phrases a sensor client will use in her mannerisms of speech include the following:

- I get a sense that...
- It seems to me that...
- What comes to me is...

Other sensor mannerisms in communication include the following:

- Client may be able to describe an awareness in general terms and, with prompting, can give more details
- Client has an elaborate story he tells that is analogous to what is happening in his body
- Client's eyes are open, and he stares intently past you or up at the ceiling
- Client looks as if he is searching for something

Questions you can ask a sensor client include the following:

- What would it like you to be aware of?
- What does it seem like to you?

You may also use a mix of audial, visual, and kinesthetic questions.

16 *Exercise Review*

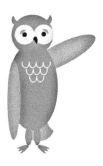

These exercises are presented throughout the book in various chapters. There are no right or wrong answers for these exercises. These answers come from client sessions and from participants of the SomaCentric Dialoguing classes. I encourage you to brainstorm and add your own. Use these answers to help you improve your dialoguing skills.

PROCESSING LANGUAGE EXERCISE
(CHAPTER 5, FRUSTRATED AARDVARKS)

How many words or phrases can you think of to indicate a client's language?

Audial	Visual	Kinesthetic	Sensor
I hear	I see	I feel	I get a sense that
it sounds like	it looks like	it feels like	It seems like
what pops into my mind is	its color/shape/ size is	it's hot/cold/ hard/soft	it wants me to know

How many questions can you ask to elicit information using a client's language?

Audial

What do you hear?

What does it sound like?

What does it want to say?

What does it want to tell you?

Visual

What do you see?

What does it look like?

What color is it?

What shape is it?

What does it want to show you?

Kinesthetic

What do you feel?

What does it feel like?

What temperature is it?

Sensor

What do you sense?

What do you notice?

What are you aware of?

What does it want you to be aware of?

ULTIMATE QUESTION/STATEMENT EXERCISE
(CHAPTER 7, OPEN-ENDED QUESTIONS VERSUS
CLOSED-ENDED QUESTIONS)

What open-ended questions or ultimate statements can you think of to elicit information?

What are you aware of?

What do you notice?

What do you sense?

Tell me what you are aware of.

Tell me more.

What is it like?

What else?

Where do you feel that? See that? Sense that? Notice that?

And…

Interesting

RESPONSES EXERCISE 1
(CHAPTER 7, OPEN-ENDED QUESTIONS VERSUS
CLOSED-ENDED QUESTIONS)

How many words can you think of that are nonjudgmental, and can be used as an appropriate response to something your client has said?

interesting	okay	good	nice
yup	yeah	uh huh	hmmmm
I hear you	Repeat back your client's own words		

"BUZZER" CEQS–OEQS EXERCISE
(CHAPTER 7, OPEN-ENDED QUESTIONS VERSUS
CLOSED-ENDED QUESTIONS)

Practice changing your questions to those that give you the most information during your dialoguing session. Let me describe to you what I do during practice sessions in my SomaCentric Dialoguing classes and individual tutoring sessions. With a group of three people, one person is the client, one is the therapist, and the third is the "buzzer." The therapist asks questions dialoguing and eliciting information from the client. The buzzer listens attentively to what is asked. Each time a question is asked that is closed-ended, leading, judgmental, or loaded, the "buzzer" makes an agreed-upon sound or signal. When the signal is given, the client will not answer the question, and the therapist asks the question in a better manner. When I am the "buzzer," I like to sit beside the therapist; each time an inappropriate question is asked, I gently poke the therapist with my finger and make a "buzzing" sound.

This helps the therapist recognize how many inappropriate questions she asks routinely. And the therapist can realize how easy it is to fall back on bad habits when it is difficult to think of open-ended questions or when the therapist experiences performance pressure. If the therapist has a difficult time rephrasing the question, the "buzzer" can offer the therapist a suggestion.

CEQS TO OEQS INTERVIEW EXERCISE
(CHAPTER 7, OPEN-ENDED QUESTIONS VERSUS
CLOSED-ENDED QUESTIONS)

Find an interview from a magazine, newspaper, or Web site. The interview must be in the format where the question is written out and then the response is written out. It can be on any subject matter. A good place to find these interviews is in the magazines by the grocery-store check-out stand (for example, *People*, *The Examiner*, *Red Book*, etc.).

For example, look for an interview that reads like this:

Q: Is it hard work being a ballerina?

A: Yes.

Q: You have done 38 productions of the *Nutcracker Suite*. I'm sure you're tired of it, aren't you?

A: Actually...

Now read through the interview. Identify which questions are closed-ended and which are open-ended. Change the closed-ended to open-ended questions that would elicit more information. If you come across a question that is leading or judgmental, change the question so that it is open-ended and not leading or judgmental.

20 QS EXERCISE
(CHAPTER 7, OPEN-ENDED QUESTIONS VERSUS CLOSED-ENDED QUESTIONS)

Find a couple of friends or colleagues to do this exercise with. Usually the game Twenty Questions is done with yes-or-no, closed-ended questions, but this exercise uses open-ended questions. The intent is to practice dialoguing and to ask questions that elicit information. Determine the length of time during which questions are asked, for example 20 minutes. One person acts as the client and chooses a subject to tell a story to the other person, the therapist. The therapist asks questions or makes statements to elicit information. The subject or story can be real or fictitious —for example, a new job, a cat gone crazy or a wild and wacky vacation.

Use open-ended questions or statements, such as "Tell me about your vacation," "Tell me more," and "How did you feel about it?" With these, the therapist elicits as much information as possible in the specified period of time. If you run out of questions before time is up, review what has been told and try to find a tangential subject about which to ask more questions to gather more information. Continue until time is up.

RESPONSES EXERCISE 2
(CHAPTER 8, WORD CHOICE)

How many words can you think of to respond appropriately to something a client has said?

Okay	Interesting	Yup
I understand	I hear you	I get that
Tell me more	Keep going	

When a client has come to a large realization I will occasionally acknowledge it with "good" or "nice" or the following:

You did some good work with that
That's a nice awareness
Beautiful   Wonderful   Wow

RELAX SYNONYMS EXERCISE
(CHAPTER 8, WORD CHOICE)

How many words can you think of to describe a state of relaxation?

soften	loosen	let go
sink	nestle	unwind
melt	wet noodle	breathe
float	lengthen	spread out
feel your arm	tighten and then let go	I'll do the work
imagine your weight	I'll hold up	let me
one step "softer"	be broad	

PAIN SYNONYMS EXERCISE
(CHAPTER 8, WORD CHOICE)

How many words can you think of that a person might use instead of the word *pain*?

pull	ache	stabbing	hot
cold	burn	numb	heavy
dull	cramp	sharp	prickly
stabbing	tight	tingly	dead
tender	empty	full	discomfort
swollen	confused	sore	dense
itchy	electrical	distracting	burning
deep	pressure	needles	feels out
dark	searing	piercing	wrenching
intermittent	draining	spasm	throbbing
cinch	shooting	out of whack	nerves firing
lack of awareness	altered sensation	irritating	

(These do not include all 38 synonyms for pain listed by *Roget's Thesaurus*.)

PROBLEM SYNONYMS EXERCISE
(CHAPTER 8, WORD CHOICE)

How many words can you think of instead of the word *problem*?

discomfort	concern	calling out	experience
awareness	situation	challenge	listen to me

STRESS SYNONYMS EXERCISE
(CHAPTER 8, WORD CHOICE)

How many words can you think of instead of the word *stress*?

| tired | harassed | can't relax | getting to me |
| wound up | tense | angry | something's off/not right |

THINK SYNONYMS EXERCISE
(CHAPTER 8, WORD CHOICE)

Think of other questions instead of "What do you think?"

What are you aware of?

What do you notice?

How is that for you?

What is your sense of that?

How do you experience that?

WIGGLE WORDS EXERCISE
(CHAPTER 9, WIGGLE WORDS)

How many more Wiggle Words or phrases can you think of?

| possibly | maybe, maybe not | perhaps |
| how about… | what if… | correct me |

How many Wiggle Word sentences can you think of?

Correct me if I'm wrong…

It seems to me…

This is what I'm hearing…

Help me out here.

Would it be fair to say that…

Let me know if I'm inaccurate…

Please let me know if this resonates with you…

JUST BECAUSE EXERCISE
(CHAPTER 12, GEMS AND NUANCES)

What other types of Just Becauses can you think of?

Pet the dog or cat

See a movie with a friend

Go to lunch with a friend

Sleep in

Take a nap

Go to a concert

Take a vacation

Eat a brownie

Take dance lessons

Buy a hat

17 *Next?*

What is next, and where do you go from here? As the saying goes, the best way to get to Carnegie Hall is "Practice, practice, practice." The same applies with the concepts and techniques of SomaCentric Dialoguing. Practice with your colleagues and friends. Do not hesitate to say to your client, "Let's try something new that I just learned." Clients love it when their therapist expands her skills, especially when it can help them resolve their situations easier.

One way to improve as a therapist is to get sessions from others who are doing SomaCentric Dialoguing. The more you experience this work, the easier it will be for you to use it with your clients. To find a therapist in your area, contact the CLEAR Institute, the organization through which SomaCentric Dialoguing workshops are taught. (See "Resources" for contact details.)

The best way to improve your understanding and SomaCentric Dialoguing skills is to take classes in SomaCentric Dialoguing. Currently, there are two levels of SomaCentric Dialoguing classes available. These classes cover the material presented in this book and more.

Another way to continue your learning is to read books on related subjects. Please see the bibliography for recommended reading.

Above all, I invite you to enhance your own learning by being creative and putting your own "thumprint" on these techniques.

GLOSSARY

Babel fish: a fictitious small, yellow fish, from the book *The Hitchhiker's Guide to the Galaxy* by Douglas Adams, which is used to translate one language to another, mentioned in chapter 5, "Frustrated Aardvarks"

Body-centered awareness: a state of being conscious of what is occurring within one's body

Closed-ended question (CEQ): a question that requires a yes-or-no answer or specific information

Communicate: to exchange information or knowledge, verbally or nonverbally

Communication language: a style of communication with distinct characteristics of thought patterns and expressions

Conversation: to use words to exchange thoughts or ideas

Deadly Words: words that carry a negative connotation or impact, words used in everyday language that can have an unseen negative effect on one's health

Dialogue: to have a meaningful communication between two parties

Facilitate: to make easy, to help and assist

Facilitator: one who helps and assists, rather than actively does

Flash-pan thoughts: thoughts or awarenesses that come as an immediate response or gut reaction to a question

Holding pattern: a place where physical restrictions frequently occur in the same manner

Indicator Compass: the manner in which a therapist is able to track or determine if something the client is saying is accurate

Knowledge: information that has been learned from a memorization of words, rather than experience

Language: a system of words used to communicate. See *communication language* and *processing language.*

Leading question: a question that suggests the answer or contains the information within the question

Loaded question: a question that contains an assumption, if the person admits to the question

No-No Words: words to avoid in dialoguing because of ambiguity (e.g., *relax, pain, problems, stress, think,* and *safe*)

Open-ended question (OEQ): a question that cannot be answered with a simple yes or no or a single piece of information

Processing language: a style of how one learns, comprehends, and interprets information

Protection: an inborn aspect of a person that keeps him or her safe

Resistance: a force or process that has the ability to oppose progress, especially when the force perceives the changes as being detrimental to itself, rather than perceiving them as being beneficial to its host

Resonance: a sympathetic vibration; people can resonate in harmony with each other

Resonate: to feel in harmony with, to feel comfortable with, to be of similar vibration or energy

Script: a phrase or series of words that are used in common language

SomaCentric Dialoguing: soma (body) centric (centered) dialoguing; a system of dialoguing with a person using her communication and processing languages in conjunction with concepts and techniques to help the person realize what her body wants her to be aware of

Somatic: pertaining to the body

SomatoEmotional Release (SER): term coined by John Upledger, DO, for a manual therapy that helps a client release emotions stored at a cellular level, by facilitating awareness of the emotions. Also used to describe the type of release that people exhibit when releasing emotions.

Talk: to communicate or have an exchange of ideas

Talking-stick rules: a concept used in Native American council meetings as a way to indicate who is allowed to speak; often indicated by holding a stick or other object

Understanding: information gathered from experience, rather than a memorization of words

Wiggle Word: a word or phrase that is used to show ownership of the thought being expressed and to indicate that what is being said may or may not be accurate

Resources

Agreement Dynamics, Inc.
Relationships, Agreements, Results
206-546-8048
800-97-AGREE
www.agreementdynamics.com
Success Signals workshops and *Success Signals*, a book by Rhonda Hilyer

CLEAR Institute
Communication, Language, Expression, Awareness, Realization—Be CLEAR!
Julie McKay, director
443-604-1981
www.clearinstitute.net
www.somacentricdialoguing.net
SomaCentric Dialoguing books and workshops
Success Signals books and workshops

Healing from the Core
Suzanne Scurlock-Durana
P.O. Box 2534
Reston, VA 20195
703-620-4509
www.healingfromthecore.com
Workshops about boundaries and grounding and *Full Body Presence*, a book by Suzanne Scurlock-Durana

BIBLIOGRAPHY

Ash, Don. *Lessons from the Sessions*. Rochester, NH: self-published, 2005.

Carson, Rick. *Taming Your Gremlin: A Surprisingly Simple Method for Getting Out of Your Own Way*. Rev. ed. New York: Quill, 2003.

———. *A Master Class in Gremlin-Taming®: The Absolutely Indispensable Next Step for Freeing Yourself from the Monster of the Mind*. New York: HarperCollins, 2008.

Dass, Ram. *Be Here Now*. Santa Fe, NM: Hanuman Foundation, 1978.

Gladwell, Malcolm. *Blink: The Power of Thinking without Thinking*. New York: Back Bay Books, 2007.

Hilyer, Rhonda. *Success Signals*. Seattle: Agreement Dynamics, 2001.

Jackson, Carole. *Color Me Beautiful*. New York: Ballantine Books, 1987.

Markova, Dawna. *The Open Mind: Exploring the 6 Patterns of Natural Intelligence*. Berkeley, CA: Red Wheel/Weiser, 1996.

McIntosh, Nina. *The Educated Heart: Professional Boundaries for Massage Therapists, Bodyworkers, and Movement Teachers*. 2nd ed. Philadelphia: Lippincott Williams and Wilkins, 2005.

Myss, Carolyn. *Anatomy of the Spirit: The Seven Stages of Power and Healing*. New York: Harmony Books, 1996.

———. *Why People Don't Heal and How They Can*. New York: Three Rivers Press, 1998.

Scurlock-Durana, Suzanne. *Full Body Presence: Healing from the Core Media*. Reston, VA: Healing from the Core Media, 2008.

Stone, Jon. *The Monster at the End of This Book* (Big Little Golden Book). New York: Golden Books, 2004.

Upledger, John. *SomatoEmotional Release and Beyond*. Palm Beach Gardens, FL: UI Publishing, 1990.

INDEX

ABOUT THE AUTHOR

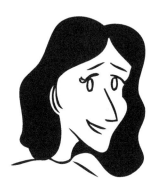

"I love what I do—providing clients with hope and the opportunity to heal the pain, trauma, and stress from their lives. Each day, I feel very honored that clients allow me the opportunity to work with them. SomaCentric Dialoguing and bodywork touch the essence of one's being. It is my privilege to hold the space for my clients to be in that place of healing."

Julie McKay, CST-D, NCTMB, BFRP, is the director of the CLEAR Institute. She is a highly respected therapist and instructor. She draws on over 20 years of experience in leadership, sales, and management and as a therapist, with a strong emphasis on communication and organization skills.

As an accomplished practitioner, Julie has a deep love for the work she does to help big and little people feel better. Julie maintains a private practice in Ellicott City, Maryland, as a Diplomate Certified CranioSacral Therapist and Nationally Certified Bodyworker, specializing in SomaCentric Dialoguing, Advanced CranioSacral Therapy, Brain Curriculum, and Lymphatic Drainage. She is also a Bach Foundation Registered Practitioner, and Enzyme Nutrition Specialist. Through Agreement Dynamics, Inc., she is a certified Success Signals presenter. Through the CLEAR Institute, Julie teaches workshops on SomaCentric Dialoguing and Success Signals communication skills.

www.JulieMcKay.net